LIVE
BEAUTIFUL

LIVE BEAUTIFUL

A COMPASSIONATE, BALANCED
GUIDE TO EVERYDAY
WELLNESS & WELL-BEING

Renée Marie

RM

Live Beautiful Publishing

COPYRIGHT © 2023 RENÉE MARIE JOYAL

LIVE BEAUTIFUL

A Compassionate, Balanced Guide to Everyday Wellness & Well-Being

ISBN	978-1-5445-3848-8	*Hardcover*
	978-1-5445-3849-5	*Paperback*
	978-1-5445-3850-5	*Ebook*
	978-1-5445-3964-5	*Audiobook*

CONTENTS

To everyone who has encouraged me to follow my dreams
and inspired me to be the person I am today.

For more information and resources, scan the QR code below to view my website, livebeautifulbook.com.

MY PASSION

My journey in the world of wellness began in my early adolescence, after alarmingly suffering a life-threatening illness. Following multiple surgeries, weeks in the ICU, and months spent in the hospital, I was told I would have to learn to adapt to my lifestyle and live with lifelong limitations. In the years that followed, I found myself forced to overcome multiple physical and mental ailments. After years of suffering through mystery health issues and countless doctors' visits, I finally received a grim prognosis with no clear direction for true healing or survival. This led me on a lifelong journey, trying every option presented to me by some of the world's best doctors. When nothing worked, I tapped into my own strength as a researcher. My findings encouraged me to experiment and create a new way of life that ultimately suppressed my symptoms and helped put my condition into remission naturally.

Health and wellness instinctively became a lifelong pursuit and passion while determinedly searching for answers to live a better life. In my research and journey to optimal health, I have naturally become an advocate in the health and wellness space, seeking a whole-body approach to both mental health and wellness.

I feel compelled to share the knowledge and research I wish I could have found when I needed it.

Adopting ayurvedic practices and creating mindful habits and rituals has not only helped me strengthen my well-being but has also created a desire and appreciation for how I choose to live in this world and enjoy every day.

WHY LIVING A BEAUTIFUL LIFE IS AN INVITATION

There are so many health books on the market, often associating with a name or label to identify themselves. My aim is to be different in offering a simple lifestyle guide to help you live a healthier, happier, and stronger life while enjoying the beauty in every day. In the last few years, wellness has become a highly dominant lifestyle value that is profoundly changing our behavior and changing the fitness and nutrition world. As we incorporate more wellness values into our daily lifestyles and become more intentional, more integrative, and more holistic, there is a renewed need for simple knowledge and education.

It is through a process of self-care habits that we can heal, flourish, and grow. The simple act of adding just one step into your daily routine can make a significant impact on your life. As novelist, poet, and thought leader Jack Kerouac said, "One day I will find the right words, and they will be simple."

I originally discovered the fundamental health strategies in this book because I had to live through them. I searched endlessly for answers to a healthier and happier life, and I wish there had been something like this for me when I needed it! My aim is to help others achieve a healthy lifestyle full of abundance. You don't have to wait until something happens to start living a healthier life. My hope is to help ease you into some of the basic concepts that helped transform my life. The benefits attained by adding just a few small lifestyle changes will perpetuate newfound strength and personal well-being.

Our world forever changed in 2020. But crisis moments also present an opportunity: more modern and flexible use of simple measures, modalities, and a revived appreciation for life's true pleasures. As we battle a global pandemic and an ever-changing, chaotic world, what better time than now to encourage a genuinely healthy lifestyle and a deeper understanding of keeping a strong mind, body, and immune system while better reorienting our relationship with ourselves; reminding ourselves that we are our own healer, and only those who make the time truly live.

LIVE BEAUTIFUL

Welcome to *Live Beautiful*. A book where you will find a combination of recipes for self-care, moments of quiet reflection, and practical steps you can take to show yourself the love and attention you sincerely deserve to achieve a beautiful life (to live "beautiful").

Living beautiful is a lifestyle, nurturing every aspect of yourself; mind, body, and spirit. This book is a lifetime book. Use this as your go-to guide to replace your habits with new, fresh, and healthier ones, finding internal balance and well-being.

You will find simple guidance and some basic knowledge through a personalized, holistic, whole-body approach that will help you:

- Feel more empowered to choose what is right for you and your lifestyle.

- Understand the nuances of the mind-body connection and of doing what makes you feel your very best each day.

- Learn to be open to both traditional and nontraditional approaches, including holistic approaches and alternative therapies.

- Bridge the gap between western and eastern medicine.

- Learn how to live organically by meeting the ever-changing demands of life.

- Appreciate that wellness is not a destination but a journey.

- Practice nurturing your inner life through preventative wellness.

- Delay symptoms of aging and diseases by adopting a healthy lifestyle.

- Heal through food and lifestyle changes.

- Learn the most effective ways to let your natural beauty shine through.

- Gain a holistic perspective on what it means to take care of yourself.

- Notice the inseparable relationship between the mind and the body.

- Luxuriate in the ever-present moment.

No matter what journey you are on, wellness all comes down to healing, and healing is building strength for life's sail.

MY STORY, MY JOURNEY

I was always healthy, happy, and active growing up. At age eleven, my life was forever changing, and I had no idea of the journey ahead of me. I remember one afternoon telling my mom I did not feel well and had a throbbing pain in my head for a couple of days. After a visit to my family physician, the doctor conducted some normal tests, and when I assumed we were done and going home, the doctor said, "Renée, enjoy your vacation." Little did I know that meant I was to be admitted to the hospital for the next ten days for treatment of a life-threatening internal staph infection of my bloodstream that was rapidly attacking my body's major organs. My brain, heart, and lungs were suddenly at risk from this invasive bloodstream infection.

By age twelve, my hormones were abruptly changing, and the first menstruation that came and never left led me to become severely anemic and in need of a blood transfusion. My body and the normal that I knew were rapidly changing. I did not feel like myself. I had no energy and felt sick every day. I had countless visits with different doctors to get my hormones and cycle under control. Finally, I was provided with labels for the condition and symptoms I had been wrestling with. At the age of thirteen, I discovered that I had PCOS.

At the forefront of my adolescence, I felt the pressure to act as normal as possible and not let symptoms or labels define me. During this discovery phase, I was striving to be just like all the other kids involved in activities and athletics, but I remained extremely lethargic and quietly in the depths of physical suffering. I was discouraged and confused, not having the energy that my peers had. I was always athletic and never wanted to show signs of weakness. Being active was an outlet for me to disengage from the reality of what I was experiencing and feel normal. It also created a self-awareness in my athletic ability to listen to my body. Something was very wrong. I began having difficulty walking up the stairs without being short of breath. I could not lay on my side without discomfort or chest pain. I lost the ability to yawn, take a deep breath, or even lay on my side. I felt as though I had an elephant on my chest.

I spent countless days meeting with doctors to help identify the root cause of these dire symptoms. Looking physically healthy on the outside, doctors explained to me this could be a hormone connection, that my chest bone was growing as I was probably experiencing symptoms of a growth spurt. I was prescribed ibuprofen to manage the symptoms and bring the inflammation down. I began taking Advil as if it came from a Pez candy dispenser. What I did *not* know was this was *not* normal. This is not how you are supposed to feel. You should not have to medicate daily. I was chronically ill, struggling, and suffering, and I did not know my body was failing me.

I struggled for one year with a constant feeling of being short of breath, assuming it was normal for a teenage girl. On a beautiful summer afternoon in June of 1999, I was at a friend's birthday party. As typical teenage girls do, we were having pizza, listening to music, and playing on a trampoline. As I took my first jump on the trampoline, I felt as though my body lost electricity. I immediately collapsed. The girls remained jumping, and I struggled to quickly remove myself from the trampoline. As I jumped off, I ran into the bathroom of my friend's house and began vomiting. Struggling for a normal breath, I called my mom to pick me up immediately. I knew something was terribly wrong. I looked normal and healthy; no one really seemed to take me seriously. Whatever was going on was invisible, but very powerful.

Nothing made sense. I had no control over what was happening. I started to lose my ability to stand, and the pressure on my chest felt like a thousand pounds. I was rushed to the hospital.

Shortly after arriving, my body shut down. I remember waking up to both of my parents speaking to a doctor with two chest x-rays illuminated on the wall. The doctor said, "This is the chest x-ray of a normal heart, and this is the x-ray of Renée's heart, which is enlarged and showing weakness in what we would see in a heart of a ninety-year-old patient. This is a life and death situation, and time is not on your side."

As the doctors hurried to supply me with oxygen, they also decided the local hospital was unequipped to handle my current health situation and ordered a helicopter to quickly Medflight me to a larger hospital in Boston. From there, everything changed. As the doctors worked to control the massive swelling in my heart, my life was no longer in my hands. I woke up to a tube in my chest, unable to walk, go to the bathroom, or function. I lost all control of my independence. I underwent surgery to drain fluid from my pericardium, the critical layer that encloses your heart and the roots of the heart's vessels, by way of a pericardial tap. Surgeons inserted a needle through the chest wall below my breastbone and into the tissue around my heart.

At age fourteen, of course, the first question I asked when I woke up was "Am I going to have a scar?" I was so nervous about my appearance, being mid adolescent. I had never even had a boyfriend. Still, I had no idea why this was happening. Why my body was failing me. In less than twenty-four hours—and without warning—I was being wheeled into another emergency and told I was going to need another surgery immediately, but I would have to be awake—I could not have anesthesia since I had just eaten my first meal. To my surprise, another pericardial tap was being inserted into the protective lining surrounding my heart. I was in excruciating pain and too weak to feel terrified. I was in and out of consciousness. I woke up at some point in the night to a priest with his hands and rosary beads on my feet. At the time, I did not understand that medically I was given my last rights. I quickly became fearful to witness a priest praying for me at my bedside. I am thankful, however, that I was at least polite when I mustered up the only energy I had and asked him to leave!

Thankfully, prayers were answered, and I was moved into recovery. I found a new residence in the hospital for the next three months. After running an exhausting battery of tests, scans, and bloodwork, and meetings with some of the world's most well-renowned heart specialists, I learned I was suffering from a life-threatening virus that had attacked my heart, or possibly an autoimmune disorder known as lupus, which was making a run for one of my major organs, my heart. My entire immune system was in disarray. I was told this would most likely be a battle that I would be fighting for the rest of my life.

This was the beginning of my journey in health and wellness. I was determined to regain my health and independence. I was finally released from the hospital and sent home with daily instructions on how to manage the pain, the flare-ups, and the tell-tale signs of more critical care with a drug treatment regimen. I had to learn to consume an unimaginable number of medications, taking multiple pills at different times daily with countless side effects. These were not the typical Flintstone vitamins I had once enjoyed! My body and joints ached, my face was flush with what is referred to as a butterfly rash, and my hair was falling out. I felt inflammation throughout my joints and body.

It was difficult to tell if the medications were helping or hindering me. With the onset of neuropathy and loss of sensation in my hands and feet, it became apparent how inflamed my central nervous system was. I began discovering new symptoms as time went on, and doctors would then prescribe me additional medication to treat my symptoms. The side effects of the medications were very real and debilitating. Operating on what felt like guesswork alone, I was entering a vicious treatment cycle while rotating between rheumatologist, cardiologist, immunologist, and endocrinologist appointments regularly.

A mystery illness is much more pervasive than conceivable. Without significant change to my health and unrelenting strong symptoms and health ailments, I was brought in for a discussion with my doctors and parents about next steps if things did not begin to get better, which was to remove the lining of my heart, known as the pericardium. Before pursuing this very dangerous option, they suggested a drug trial that could help but had serious side effects that could cause cancer and infertility.

The suggested steps were nothing I was able to accept. I should be going to school and preparing for college. How could I, and why would I take a drug that would cause such damage to my body? How could I make myself healthier? What steps could I take to heal and protect myself? It was from this moment that I sought out change and relentlessly pursued healing myself by combining eastern and western medicine.

With word circulating about my health, an expert alternative medicine doctor contacted me. Hearing of my story, he said, "I am a healer, and I want to help heal you holistically." He amazed me by reaching out, and insistently refused payment for any treatment. He said, "See if this helps—and if we can get your nervous system functioning properly and your body in alignment to better defend itself."

Deep down, I knew my only hope in attacking this virus was a strong immune system. While the medications I was prescribed were critical for my care at the time, they were also strongly suppressing my immune system.

Meeting this alternative medicine doctor had offered me hope and insight into healing my body. From that vantage point, he gave me perspective and knowledge to help strengthen my immune system holistically.

The doctor taught me ways to reduce nervous system disruption, and how health can return to my body—things you do not hear in typical conventional medicine.

The combination of both conventional and alternative treatments began to show a significant reduction in my symptoms, and my body was responding. Committed to strengthening my immune system as if I were preparing for war, I was able to slowly decrease the heavy doses of medications. Within six to twelve months of adopting a healthy lifestyle and alternative modalities, my body responded incredibly. My last-resort surgery and need for medication treatment with cancer-causing side effects were no longer on the table! I was finally making a turn to control this mystery illness.

MY LIFE NOW

I became a collector of information. This disease did not come out of thin air. There were tell-tale signs early on that a virus could have damaging effects on my body and nervous system.

I could not accept the fact that I had to feel bad each day and prepare myself for future health issues that autoimmune diseases often dictate. I never wanted to put limitations on what I could or could not do. Never settling for a simple answer, I spent countless years trying to self-heal and educate myself, not only to prevent health issues but to feel my very best in any way I could. I accepted the diagnosis of autoimmune disease, but refused to accept the prognosis of a life defined by it.

The result of days and nights of countless research defied my doctor's expectations. Today, I proudly remain in remission and have no sign of PCOS or lupus. While autoimmune diseases such as lupus remain dormant in the body, I have been able to listen to my body and maintain control of my symptoms. I am not defined by an illness. I am defined by my health and what I can control.

I have taken preemptive steps through nutritional and lifestyle changes, and I have been able to prevent further health issues and live a beautiful life. Medical science could not give me answers or an explanation about why I had an autoimmune disease, or how I could heal from it. I was simply provided with a tag, not an answer.

MY MISSION

To empower people to become their healthiest, happiest, most authentically beautiful selves while supporting the enjoyment of an aligned, balanced, sustainable, and deeply gratified way of life.

There is always an opportunity each day to make a positive difference. Your balanced and beautiful life begins here...

CHAPTER 1

THE PATH TO GRATITUDE

*"Gratitude is the fairest blossom
which springs from the soul."*

—Henry Ward Beecher

GRATITUDE

With each new life and each new day comes a new meaning. Every day, every person, and every *body* is different, and that is uniquely beautiful. Not one day, not one person, not one moment is the same. Some people may have moments of déjà vu, which is the closest opportunity we have to live the same moment twice, but every moment is different and brings new meaning. That new meaning is personal to each and every one of us, and what you make of it is down to you.

Most of the human race seems to take life for granted. It can become an easy routine and way of life to wake up each day without being thankful for the fresh start and opportunities that are available. For most people, it takes a certain turn of events to realize that they need to cherish life more and stop taking it for granted. Once you come to that realization, your mindset can easily change by taking the small steps laid out in this book—learning to live beautiful. From the moment we wake up, we can—and should—feel grateful. We can open our eyes to a new day and see it as a new journey, a new healthy path. Not only should we be grateful, but we should also consistently practice gratitude.

Waking up healthy and happy is a blessing we all take for granted at times. At age twenty-five, I reached what I had thought was an insurmountable goal in my wellness journey. I was finally healthy, strong, symptom-free, and my autoimmune disease diagnosis had remarkably reached remission.

Only months later, on a cold, dreary winter evening, my life quickly shifted in a matter of seconds. I became a survivor, fighting for my life as a passenger in a nearly fatal drunk driving accident that turned my life upside down.

Only five minutes away from home, I found myself screaming for my life until my voice ran out. I was certain the tractor-trailer headlights staring straight at me would be the last image I would see before my time on earth was up. Within a fraction of a second, the vehicle I was in collided with the semitruck. I was pinned underneath an eighteen-wheeler, in shock, fully conscious, while the driver remained comatose and

THE PATH TO GRATITUDE

in an unknown state. Only inches away from being severed, I was unable to move as the vehicle had nearly collapsed like an accordion on top of me. I screamed with the only voice I could force to raise, but no one would come towards the vehicle, frightened of what they would see or if an explosion would ensue. After waiting for what felt like an eternity for first responders to arrive, I was finally removed from the vehicle by what firefighters call the "jaws of life." Still uncertain of the driver's survival or condition, I found myself on my way to a hospital once again.

By chance, I miraculously escaped with minor bodily trauma, but in the months ahead, the mental trauma would be my biggest battle. In a relentless effort to cherish life and live fully, I began the journey of writing my own self-care prescription—turning my pain into purpose.

Feeling as though my body had been through war, my autoimmune disease was beginning to take force, reactivating once again.

Fear triggers many changes. I knew I was granted a second chance at life. I began making choices—who to share my life with, how to use my time, and how to live a quality, healthy life with the time I am gifted. I had to make a choice to be unaffected by the turbulence of my current situation. I dove deeper beyond diet and nutrition to fully enhance my well-being. Feeling grateful for life and what it means to be truly alive, I put in the work, letting go of attachments, increasing my perspective, and living more deeply in the present moment.

Life is precious, and our time is not guaranteed. Had I not fought so hard for health in my previous years, I do not know if my mind and body would have been so well primed for life's unexpected hardships. I am forever grateful for the work I had previously devoted to keeping my body strong and conditioning my mind to bear life's unforeseen obstacles. I could have looked at this reckless drunk driving nightmare as a major setback in my health journey, but my mind would not allow me to reflect negatively for one second. I have so much gratitude for life and the chance I have to fight for it every day! How we adapt and respond to challenges and the mindset we approach life with makes all the difference. No day should be wasted. I am forever grateful to be here to reinforce the power of gratitude and what it can do for you.

It is easy to take little things for granted and let time dictate our ability to care for ourselves. Let's work together to change that mindset. Not only are we in control of our lives, but we are also in control of our thoughts and attitude. Small moments that are special can slip through our fingers too easily. These small moments, with every other moment, should be cherished. If you make each new meaning powerful and purposeful, then your outlook on life can change.

Practicing a life you want is your choice. Being in control is a blessing. Manifesting a beautiful, quality life is possible. Let's get started.

IN A WORLD WHERE YOU CAN
BE ANYTHING, BE KIND

Don't you agree that the world would be a better place if we were all kind to one another? Practicing being kind is one of the easiest starting points in this journey, both for yourself and others. If you show kindness, others are more likely to show it back. Even the smallest of gestures can positively impact not only yourself but also those around you.

The easiest way to put this rule into action is as simple as thinking before you speak or act. Begin by practicing this and testing the outcome on those closest to you. Most people are naturally comfortable showing emotion to close friends and family, so trying this on them is a good place to start.

The next time you're in conversation with a close friend or family member, think about what you want to say before speaking the words. Often, the human instinct is to speak as soon as possible to get your word in. Hold off instead, and think calmly about what you want to say. The more you practice taking your time to think before speaking, the more natural it will feel. Before you know it, you will do it without even realizing it. These small steps are important to change your gratitude and actions towards others and become a better version of yourself.

You will most likely notice a change in tone and pace too. The way you address a person is just as important as what you say. Think about your body posture and tone of voice when having a conversation. Relaxed expressions, both bodily and facially, reflect a kind manner.

Passing on this mindset is even easier. Once you are kind to those close to you, those skills will manifest into them. They will then pass on this practice to others. The beneficial enhancement is unprecedented. Kindness filters through, and if we can all learn to be kind to others, then this mindset can spread as far as we wish.

The beautiful thing about being kind is that it is instinctual. We are all born with emotional needs, and the way we use our emotions is down to us. We just need to put the positive emotions into practice more.

Now that you have acknowledged how tone of voice and expression can help you practice and address kindness, next is the mental attitude towards yourself. Yes, being kind to others is important, but it is just as important to be kind to yourself.

Listening to what your body wants and needs is something we don't do often enough. Cultivating sensory awareness is critical. Letting your body rest when it needs to, filling it with delicious, nutritious foods, stretching, and practicing mindfulness is a good place to start. Optimize your time so that you have an hour or two daily to nourish your body and your mind. Be kind to yourself, and your soul will appreciate it and feel fulfilled, which is necessary to practice and enhance gratitude. Thus, doing something kind for yourself can create a ripple effect, and is attainable for anybody.

PRACTICING COMPASSION

Going out of your way for others is not only reflecting on your kindness but is also practicing compassion. Thinking out of the box and out of your own emotions to focus that energy on the physical and mental emotions of others is powerful.

First, we must learn to empathize with others. While most of us think we practice compassion in every circumstance, it may not always be the case. We may sometimes disregard the mental or emotional pains of others since they aren't visible. Not being able to physically see a peer's pain can sometimes make us think it isn't true or serious. But mental pain can be more consequential than physical. Your peer could be suffering more than you could ever know because you are unable to observe the pain.

The best way to practice compassion is to use your imagination. Think of a time you were in mental pain and imagine your closest friend going through that. You would want to help them, wouldn't you? You would feel empathy and want to do anything you could to pull them out of that pain.

And that is exactly what compassion looks and feels like: empathizing with others to help them overcome bad times in their life.

On the flip side, being honest with yourself is a way to practice self-compassion. At times, we may disregard our own emotions. We may feel sad and avoid reacting to them. It is important to learn to forgive yourself and not be harsh on yourself. Avoiding your emotions will only make them build up and become toxic. Express yourself, express your gratitude, and be mindful. Employing a growth mindset will help you balance your self-compassion, learn to deal with your emotions, and grow your self-love. Beauty is an expression of soul, not ego. When we focus on the good things we enjoy in life, we have more to live for and tend to take better care of ourselves.

Move through life with grace, honesty, and compassion, and learn to live beautiful. You will not regret it.

OPEN HEART

How can I serve today? There is always an opportunity each day to make a positive difference.

Make your heart the most beautiful thing about you.

Everyone's journey in life is unique, but we are all trying to reach the same destination—a beautiful one. How we direct our attention to our health, our energy, our diet, and the people we surround ourselves with—how we choose to spend our incredibly precious time—are all part of that unique journey. Health and well-being aren't just about our bodies but also about our minds and our behavior.

By nurturing your ability to live intentionally, venturing beyond the usual routine, you create opportunities to gain a new, fresh perspective. When you change your thinking pattern and realign yourself, you can raise your frequency and attract so much more into your life.

Take the first step in a direction that feels right. Know that time is precious and nonrefundable. Where we choose to focus our time and energy is essential in cultivating a quality life full of abundance.

The mind and the body are so intertwined that by immersing yourself in the place of non-judgment with an open heart, you inherently increase the quality of your relationships, community, and connection. It is the true catalyst for wellness in relationships of all kinds. Making yourself vulnerable to everyday life and challenges will serve as a beneficial enhancement and help you live in the moment.

Design your life and a way to share it with the world. It's amazing how fluid and effortless your life and everyday reality can be when your worldview shifts. Realize how much your life improves when you have an open heart.

There are three obligatory rules for learning to be nonjudgmental and keeping your heart open: understand, accept, and love. Learning to be thankful for life and expressing your gratitude comes with not judging others, or yourself for that matter. Cultivate nonjudgmental awareness, free from bias or critique. Too often, we judge people too quickly. The next time you find yourself unconsciously about to judge someone, engage your senses and put these three rules into action.

Understand

There is a quote by American poet Walt Whitman that we should all stand by: "Be curious, not judgmental." Something as simple as that puts this rule into perspective. Instead of focusing your energy on judging someone, take a step back and try to be curious; try to understand the person and put yourself in their shoes. Think about where they might come from, what their life holds—or better yet, ask them. Being curious about someone and even striking up a conversation will help you avoid passing judgment.

We must understand that everyone is different. Everyone has a different story, different reason(s), and a different outlook on life. We all choose to live life differently. We all choose our own paths. Taking a step back and losing your judgment will not only better you as a person but will help you practice gratitude and mature your outlook. If you saw someone judging you, you probably wouldn't like it. It might make you feel self-conscious or unconsciously lower your self-esteem. The same goes for others if you judge them. Imagine how it would make them feel. Be understanding and be curious.

Accept

After you've understood (or tried to understand) the person, the next step is acceptance. If you can understand a person and why they are the way they are, accepting them is a big part of being nonjudgmental.

Accepting someone for who they are shows you are inclusive and receptive. It shows you are not trying to change them—that you have understood and welcomed their story and their meaning.

The acceptance stage is probably the hardest part for some. But once you understand that the world just is what it is—and that *it is*, for the most part, unchangeable—you can learn to accept it. The same can be said for the people in it. Otherwise, the only thing you will obtain is frustration. Focus on the good, even if it is only your increased sensory knowledge. In today's paradigm, control of life belongs to awareness. There is something to learn from everyone.

Your soul is the most intimate part of you. The only part of the world you can and need to change is you. Choosing not to judge others and accepting people for who they are will better you as a person. It will deepen your understanding of the world, its being, and its meaning.

Love

Understanding and accepting people for who they are will make you love people's individual qualities. Not only that, but it is also a form of self-love and self-appreciation.

This universal truth stands, loving others will help them love others (like ripples in a pond). It will also help them love themselves. This love chain will continue and grow the more you accept and love others for who they are. This love can create a positive ripple effect and, eventually, extend further than you ever imagined. It will filter through the world and, hopefully, make the world a more loving place.

It is always better to share the love and pass on positive vibes. When you act with unconditional kindness and compassion, you can enhance the overall well-being of yourself and others. The more love you share, the faster it will expand. Teach someone these rules, and you won't be the only one practicing gratitude. Put simply, you cannot live your most fulfilling life without opening your heart.

BE YOUR OWN TEACHER

The beautiful thing about being you is that you can be your own teacher. You can teach yourself new things, new strengths, and practices better than anyone else can. You can listen to your mind and your body to feel and know what it wants. You know best what areas of life you need to focus on improving, and what new things you can put into place to be a better version of yourself.

Make kindness towards yourself and others a daily habit! Having the ability to teach yourself something new every day is powerful. You can practice whatever you want when you want. Being organized and motivated to teach yourself new things comes with having a daily schedule and routine. You can teach yourself something new by incorporating a little bit each day. It is the microsteps that often create the largest life-enhancing results, and it will soon become a part of you. You can cultivate new action patterns.

For instance, if you want to learn a new language, give yourself thirty to sixty minutes every day to have a lesson. Fitting this time into your daily schedule will soon become routine, and this skill will develop. Being your own teacher means you can fit this time into your day anywhere that suits you. There are no rules in the school of self-development.

We all have the opportunity to manifest the life we want and control our own lives, so start now. There's no need to delay teaching yourself new skills, as it is you who is in charge of your day and what you choose to fill it with.

If you have other responsibilities that need attention, make sure you take responsibility for yourself too. You are the change agent. The only person who can better you is you. The only person who can organize your time is you.

Be honest and open with people who place demands on your time. Everyone is understanding as they all need it too. Telling your family or friends that you are learning a new skill or dedicating time for self-enhancement may encourage them to do the same, which will help elicit positivity for deepening your pursuit of good in the world. This can help you and your peers develop gratitude for the ability to continue to learn, and put your exciting new skills and interests into practice.

We have to understand that the vibrancy of a beautiful life does not just happen. It has to be created with intent. Knowledge is power, and you best believe that new knowledge comes from being your own teacher.

EVERY DAY IS A GIFT

The theme here is waking up and recognizing every day as a blessing. As the saying goes, "Treat every day as a gift, that is why it is called the present." You may question why. The answer is simple. We don't do it enough.

It may sound like a big effort to practice this every morning, but cultivating gratitude in life whenever we can is important for our happiness. So why not start as soon as we wake up? Starting a day on a positive note will usually result in having a positive day.

Think of life as a plant. The moment it sees its first sign of sunshine every day, it starts to grow. For people, it's the same. The moment we wake up to a new day, we can grow, just like a plant. Putting gratitude into action can give you perspective and instantly shift your outlook on life.

Seeing every day as a gift can be practiced simply by continuing to learn and appreciating the fact that each day can bring new opportunities. Appreciating your new day will help you appreciate your life. It will help you grow, and it will help you enhance your gratitude power.

HARNESS THE POWER TO CREATE
GOOD IN THE WORLD

Show gratitude. Gratitude is not just in a journal. It is how you show up in life! Sharing your new mindset with others will help the world be a better place. Once you feel confident that you have harnessed the power and understanding of gratitude, feel confident to share the journey with others.

Little things can often bring the most happiness. Sharing your positive reactions, strengths, and knowledge on your journey will rub off on others. Being a positive and powerful person can have a pay-it-forward spirit of giving and will most likely encourage others to do better. By aligning our emotional awareness, we can enrich our lives and the world around us.

When people are around a negative person or toxic atmosphere, that energy transcends boundaries. Whatever energy you surround yourself with will affect your mood, just as it does for other people. Therefore, sharing positive emotions will enhance other people's moods, and help them practice and experience what you have and feel.

MAKE HEALTHY CHOICES AND HEALTHY HABITS

Gratitude is linked directly to your health, and making healthy choices is key to moving forward with your journey and improving your well-being.

In addition to gratitude, three areas to improve on through healthy choices are your diet, exercise routine, and quality of sleep. A healthy combination of these will enhance your energy and mood, which will later benefit you emotionally and socially.

Eating balanced, nutritious food helps energize your body, detoxify, and maintain physical strength. If you love food, there is a whole section on it later, which will help you better align your body and nourish it as you grow through the different seasons of your life.

Getting into a regular exercise routine will help enhance your mood and body. Listen to what your body wants in terms of exercise and go with the flow. Gentle exercise is just as effective as intense exercise, so discover what your body wants from working out. You may even like to change up your workouts every time you do one. Whatever you want and need is what will be best for you.

After balancing your diet and exercise routine, getting good sleep may come naturally. But, if you are a workaholic or seem to lack the motivation to prioritize sleep, make sure you switch off and get the hours you need. A fatigued body will quickly lead to an unbalanced mind and may encourage you to make bad lifestyle choices. Getting enough sleep is good practice for looking after yourself. Seven to eight hours per night is essential, and your body, mind, and soul will thank you for it.

Learning to be a better version of yourself and changing your outlook on life takes more work than just thinking you'd like to see change. You need to act on it. You have the opportunity to undertake greater effort with simple lifestyle changes that feel natural to you.

Once you've mastered your own power, you can easily pass it on to others. The way you present yourself and offer yourself to others may encourage them to go on the same journey as you. Although each person's journey will be different, the outcome will be the same and result in more people wanting to be the best version of themselves and make the world a better, more positive, and beautiful place.

Inside each of us is a beautiful soul, and we've all just got to let it free.

CHAPTER 2

LIFESTYLE

"Your present circumstances don't determine where you can go; they merely determine where you start."
—Nido Qubein

YOUR LIFELONG HOME

No matter what, there will always be external events that we have no control over. What you do have control over is what you choose to do about it. Lifestyle is the most powerful change we can make. Dig deep within yourself. Visualize the life you want. Make changes, if needed, and remember you are in control of your happiness, your state of mind, and your daily life. Time is not refundable. Use it with intention. If you are not enjoying every day, change it!

Beauty is an energy you carry; it is what you exude and radiate when you are feeling good. Your vitality is a reflection of how you choose to live. Your lifestyle, routine, and daily actions are a huge part of what make you who you are and how you feel each day. You need to start listening to yourself. You need to practice and trust what you already know to pursue a healthy, radiating, beautiful life. To do this, you need to start somewhere. Even if that somewhere is small, those small steps can turn into big, unexpected, flourishing outcomes. Often the smallest steps bring the biggest life rewards.

Nurture your body. Listen to your body. The very best investment you can make is in your own health. The most meaningful thing you can aim for is your full potential. Increase your subjective well-being and enhance your life. You are the only living being who can ultimately control your life, your time, and where you devote your energy. Setting boundaries and practicing a schedule that will help you strive to be your best self will lead to great things.

Wellness is deeply individual. How you live can be the culprit and the cure. A holistic approach to wellness is practicing total body care. Nurturing your mind will, in turn, nurture your health and improve the quality of your life. You can control how you live. Simple well-being practices are easy to integrate into your daily routine. You just need to begin.

Your body is truly the only permanent place you must live. Invest in your body and mind as if they were the foundation of your home because, in many ways, they are.

There is no need to overcomplicate or put undue pressure on yourself. There is, however, a need to give yourself the space to cultivate a beautiful life, living healthy and positive! Fitting in time to improve small areas of your life will eventually come together as one, and it will nourish and balance your entire being, increasing your health. Sometimes the most basic things have the deepest impact on our lives. These small practices will soon become a part of you, and that is when you achieve a better version of yourself. To live a truly beautiful life, you must make a commitment to yourself to feel better, be better, and live better.

How exactly do you get there? Where do you start? How do you achieve a whole body of prosperity? Let this section be your personalized blueprint. Read carefully, let this be the start of your daily practice, and use it as you step towards living beautiful.

BUILD A STRONG ROUTINE

Affirm

First stop. Happiness. The Dalai Lama said that "happiness is the highest form of health." But where do we begin? Create an affirmation for yourself—a mantra to remember and repeat every morning to start the day off right—something you believe and that resonates deep within.

Visualize

Starting the day off positively and on a good note is a big part of a balanced wellness routine. The way you start your day deeply impacts how your day will proceed. Your thoughts create your life. Visualize how you want your day to go. Make an intentional effort to be happier. Exercise your prerogative to stay healthy, happy, vibrant, and thriving; making that commitment to yourself will impact others.

Journal

The key thing to remember about journaling is that there is no right way to do it. You do not have to do it every day, and your entries certainly do not need to be compelling, beautifully written essays detailing the inner workings of your mind. A list of things you are grateful for is sufficient, as is a full-fledged rant. The point is to express yourself in a way that feels cathartic, and only when you feel compelled to do so. My journal oscillates from poetry to reflective quotes to simple thoughts, goals, and intentions, and sometimes I go for weeks without writing. I never force it.

Routine

A morning practice teaches you to go about your day positively; it is the very beginning of your daily routine. There is a secret of success to be found in your daily routine. Implement a daily routine that will nourish all aspects of your life. Do something good for your body, your soul, and your mind.

Ritual

Think of something you do—or would like to do—when you start your day; call it a ritual. This ritual should be your selfish habit, and you should practice it every day. Don't limit yourself—you can have more than one. Small but easy rituals can support calmness and clarity. Let this be something that relaxes you to set your tone for the day. Practicing something that makes you happy will keep your mind sharp and focused; it will feel like a reward. Starting your day with a sense of purpose and accomplishment will not only help you achieve great things but support you in handling derailments that life sometimes (more often than not) throws our way. The idea is to take the time to look inward. The point is not so much the activity itself as it is the ritualized reflection.

Schedule

Understandably, you will want to base your schedule around daily pressures and demands, such as work, family, and everyday obligations. That is okay, provided you fit yourself and your inner personal needs around it. Optimizing your time will allow you to be more present in the moment, and help you be more consistent. However, consistency is not necessarily key. If one day you want to avoid routine and be free, then so be it. Listen to the messages your body is sending to you, and be responsive.

Write

When you are building your new routine, write it down. Having something written down will encourage you to stick by it. Working through a to-do list can be so satisfying. Put that same method into practice with your daily schedule. Align your time to what is important, and the rest will fall into place.

Understand that time is precious. It is irrecoverable. The simple truth is we will never have today again. Nobody can order your day; only you can do that. Be in control of your life, your energy, and your time. You cannot necessarily control the way each day goes. But what you can do is decide how you want to start and end it. How you start and end your day will determine how everything else goes in between. Let's take a closer look at these steps to build a beautiful lifestyle.

SEIZE THE DAY

Wake up your mind in a BEAUTIFUL way and set the intention of positivity for your day.

Your thoughts create your life. You must think positive thoughts. When you wake up in the morning, you cannot just wait to see what kind of day you will have. You have to decide what kind of day you will have. How you start the day sets the tone for the rest of it. When you start your day with intention and routine, you create momentum for the rest of the day. So why not do something good for yourself each morning?

Starting your day on the right foot can lift your mood, get you focused, clear your head, and set you in the right direction to determine how the rest of your day will go. Your personal health begins first thing in the morning, and a few simple steps can make up your perfect morning routine.

Sunlight before Screen Light

Create tech boundaries. In a world increasingly dependent on technology, it is now more challenging than ever to place necessary limitations on our devices. The thing about the smart tech generation is that many see it as their main priority. If you find yourself opening your eyes, rolling over, and reaching for your TV, computer, or smartphone: STOP! Adding silence before catching up with news, social media, and anything over yourself is key to good mental health.

Stop and think back to the times your parents, grandparents, and the older generations would wake up and have no choice but to soak up the morning sunlight. The simple technology-free times were when natural light was the first thing the eyes would see and adjust to. Your phone can wait an extra ten minutes. Appreciate the moment, and use that time to wake up, embrace the silence, adjust your focus, and think your own thoughts.

Natural light stimulates the body's natural circadian rhythm. Instead of reaching for your phone, reach for the blinds, and let in the natural light. If you have the ability, get outside in the morning for two to ten minutes of natural light exposure and invigorate your mind and body while suppressing depressive symptoms. Your own thoughts and opinions matter more than those of others on your timeline. You are the controller of your time and actions, so let your phone rest, set the tone for your day, and appreciate the stillness of the morning.

Hydration

After a night's rest, your body loses a lot of the previous day's hydration. Your body naturally loses water, and we all wake up dehydrated. While waking up to natural light, grab yourself some water. Drinking plenty more throughout the day is key, so why not start your day by rehydrating your body. It is a great way to flush toxins from your body, boost your immune system, reduce aging, and much more. Drink your water with some lemon, lime, mint, or citrus to enhance its benefits. Citrus water is a great way to get your digestive system moving. Practice what you preach, and begin your day the way you want the rest of it to go. Elevate your water with trace mineral drops, liquid zinc, or chlorophyll drops to enhance the benefits of hydration.

Morning Motivation

There is nothing quite like a sweet cup of something in the morning. Whether that be tea, coffee, juice, or something even more life-enhancing, like a cup of matcha, get in your morning motivational brew. Make it a part of your day that you will look forward to. Slow down and thoughtfully sip to fully enjoy a unique, self-indulgent moment. While drinking and enjoying your morning cup of coffee, tea, or whatever you like, take it as a bit of time to plan your day. This is a great opportunity to map out your day, journal, make a to-do list, or simply sip and enjoy a moment to just be still. It is a great excuse to have a "me moment." Your body will function better with the right energy, and that is exactly what you need to stay focused and motivated.

Meditation

You can meditate at any time of the day, but morning meditation will help set the prospective mood for the day. It will help you focus, reenergize, and feel content and optimistic. Aim for ten minutes each day. Even if you only have time for two minutes, take it! It allows you to be mindful and focus on a particular thought, activity, or feeling and dive deep into your soul. Realize deep within yourself that the present moment is all you need and all you must control. An open, interested, and inquiring mind comes from meditation, and the practice is a great way to put your head straight if you get out of the bed on the wrong side. If you practice meditation frequently, it will train your awareness and enable you to achieve a mentally calm state. Regular practice will also help you integrate responsibility into your life and put it into practice in other areas. Meditation methods and routines will be discussed later if you are looking for guidance or want an insight into how to practice more frequently.

Get Outside

Natural light stimulates your circadian rhythm. Our circadian rhythm is a natural internal process that regulates our sleep-wake cycle daily. It repeats every twenty-four hours, and keeping it balanced can improve your physical, mental, and emotional well-being. Sitting outside first thing in the morning motivates us, and helps our body refresh as it takes in natural air. There is something infinitely healing and calming about the outside world. Starting your day with a calming moment can set the tone for the day. Taking your morning coffee, water, or meditative moment outside (or simply opening the shades) allows you to accomplish two morning practices simultaneously.

Make No Excuses

Never believe in making excuses. If you feel rushed in the morning and think you cannot manage to fit in a simple routine or even your favorite morning beverage, then you should make time. Prioritize yourself and never make excuses that are not necessary. It is too easy to make excuses for yourself. Believe me, I have been there. Yes, it is easy to stay in bed for an extra fifteen minutes, and sometimes you may need it, but dedicating your time to improving yourself and getting up an extra fifteen minutes early can change your entire day. Focus on yourself and find something you look forward to. Slowly sipping on your favorite beverage in the morning before you start your day can create a meditative moment. Once you begin making these small changes, your body will soon crave the positive, cathartic benefits. Every day is a new beginning. Treat each day as a way to master being a healthier you.

EAT RIGHT

Real Food

Feeding your body the right food will make it appreciate you. Nourish your body with whole, nutrient-rich, real foods daily—foods to optimize and enhance your health—foods that are packed with nutrients and antioxidants that support your health, vitality, and well-being.

Real food is whole, unprocessed, and natural—foods that are free from harmful chemicals, preservatives, additives, and processed sugars. Basically, limit your consumption of anything that comes from a box, can, or a jar. Use as few things as possible that come out of a package, and you will be surprised how much better you can feel. Stay as close to nature as possible. Think fruits, veggies, whole grains, nuts, eggs, meats, and fish. Eating a diet rich in nutritious, unprocessed foods has major health benefits that will enhance your body's natural defenses, improving digestion, lowering inflammation, and reducing disease risk.

Following a diet based on real food may be one of the most valuable things you can do to sustain good health and a beautiful, quality life. The things we eat and drink have a direct effect on our well-being. The word *diet* has a pernicious assumption. It is not advised to stick to a strict diet, as restricting your body from foods can only cause your happiness to decline and promote a lack of motivation. Food is meant to be enjoyed. Simply focus on eating more real foods and less processed foods through appropriate balance and intuitive eating. Don't deprive yourself. Become more conscious. Make concerted choices to live better and feel beautiful.

Food gives us life, and it's a lifestyle change that's worth the effort! Put your health and body first. Your self-care journey starts now. By nourishing your body with nutrient-rich foods, you know you are nurturing your body from the inside out. Choose to eat quality food as an act of self-love, knowing you are fueling your body to be strong, resilient, and beautiful. Real food is just one component of a self-love diet and healthy lifestyle. It's also important to get plenty of exercise, lower your stress levels, and maintain proper nutrition. We will dive deep in later chapters on the lifestyle enhancements and benefits, but there's no doubt that upgrading your diet and eating more real food will go a long way toward improving your health and well-being.

Adaptogens

Also known as functional supplements, adaptogens are nontoxic plants that help the body combat stressors. Picture them as a mini vacuum for stress. There are many you can easily integrate into meals, such as ginseng, goji berries, turmeric, and holy basil. Giving your body the right foods and added nutrients will encourage you to stay on track. Integrating adaptogens into your daily diet is key for balancing stress and hormones.

You are embarking on a journey to becoming your best self—physically and mentally. With moderation and a greater focus on intuitive eating, you will nourish your body and nourish your soul. Listen to your body throughout the day; feed it the right nutrients and fuel it needs to stay on track.

CREATE BALANCE

Prioritize

Everyone has busy lives in their own way. Whether it be due to personal requirements, family, work tasks, or life moving quickly, each and every one of us has something that keeps us occupied. Each day brings new challenges, and prioritizing is a great way to tackle and balance what is most important. If your days are getting filled up with tasks that attract you away from investing in yourself, assemble priorities and work through the tasks at a more manageable pace. This can be anything from simply learning to say no, to selecting dedicated time or days to turn off and disconnect, to creating alone time, enhancing your natural-born creativity. Not only will this help you work more thoroughly, but it will also create time for yourself, which can offer a tremendous boost in your overall happiness. Below, I share ways in which you can prioritize and cultivate new action patterns without sacrificing your valuable time.

Divide

Keeping a balance between work life and personal life is imperative for growth in both areas. If you dedicate too much time to work, it can impact your mood. Stress and being overworked can prevent you from working to your full potential. Whereas a clear head can help you give something your full effort. Having a clear mind comes with balance. Dividing your workload can benefit your personal life and give you time to work on you. Do something for yourself, and better your well-being. Time batching and blocking are good techniques to avoid dedicating too much time to one area, daily chore, or project.

Schedule

A timed routine can help you stay on track and tackle what you wish to accomplish each day. Establishing a productive routine begins with a schedule—one where you find enjoyment is vital to achieving a productive and successful day. While prioritizing a schedule may sound like work, the benefit of the time you will save in the long run is well worth the added effort. The time gained in creating a schedule and routine can allow for more self-indulgent moments that you may have never found the time for before. Not to mention the act of prioritizing your time will also aid in reducing stress levels and support your own mental wellness.

Start small by setting yourself up for a positive and productive day by adding nonnegotiables to your schedule such as one minute of breathwork, a thirty-second cold blast shower, creating time limits on your phone, making time to enjoy your morning beverage, getting outside, filling up a water pitcher to ensure you are staying hydrated throughout the day, and blocking off time for a workout of your choosing. Whatever it may be, adding these small steps as a nonnegotiable part of your daily schedule will create balance, increased health, and vitality. Once you begin adding these microsteps, you will be surprised how much your body will crave them!

Your lifestyle is a result of daily choices. Taking the time to set the tone of your day is really so important. Making space and priority to incorporate stress-relieving activities into your wellness routine like meditation, yoga, journaling, or simply taking time for a walk can really improve the quality of your life.

Creating balance is a major mind and mood stabilizer. The act of creating balance is easier said than done, as it does require a little self-discipline. You must manage yourself, not time. Build a routine that you desire. The most important thing is to find what works best for you and your lifestyle. As the author Catherine Pulsifer described, "Time and balance, the two most difficult things to have control over, yet they are both the things that we do control." Set an intention with moderation in mind. Get clear on your purpose and do it in a way that feels true and authentic to you, separating work, family, and personal time as best you can.

Schedule breaks, make daily to-do lists, have something you crave and look forward to each day, whether it be watching your favorite show, having a delicious meal, or listening to your favorite wind-down playlist. Not only will you find enjoyment, but you will intuitively stabilize the stress hormone cortisol, thus creating a healthier you! Start becoming more conscious of how you manage your time and watch your whole life change.

Creating a balanced life for yourself is just as important as balancing it for your family; your positive actions will influence those who surround you. If your family and friends see that you are taking action to live a more positive life, they will likely want to follow in your footsteps. If a new lifestyle and routine make you shine, other people will want to shine with you. Your effectiveness will inevitably inspire others. Do not forget how much influence you can have on other people, and making that influence a positive one can make those around you better people too. A little bit of life balance goes a long way.

RELAX THE DAY AWAY

We covered morning routines and affirmations. So, it is only right to work on your evenings. Ending your day positively is just as important as beginning it positively. Bookend your day. Set the pace and tone. What happens in between is greatly influenced by the beginning and end.

Stop

Finishing off your day, an activity, or a chore with some relaxation, both physically and mentally, can flush away the weight of stress on your shoulders and in your mind. So, take a momentary reprieve and delight yourself. We too easily get caught up in the everyday hustle and forget that life is precious, and we need to pause and take time to be good to ourselves.

Switch Off

Relaxing your mind, body, and spirit comes with being present in the moment. If you want to practice relaxation, my biggest tip is to do it in the evenings. When you switch off from work or finish a task and have free time, it is your choice how you fill it.

Tech NO

Free time may seem like a chance to switch off from work and switch on technology. Technology cannot give back to you like real conversation, exercise, and mindfulness can. You may feel that being present in the moment is being online with other people, but there is nothing more present than being in the moment with yourself, your loved ones, and the things you love in real time.

Start an evening ritual and create an ideal environment. Unwind. Relax your mind whenever you get the chance to. Create a wind-down routine. Turn off the tech, dim the lights, cue the music or white noise, and light some candles or diffuse essential oils. Taking time for self-care can be a nice transition between screens and sleep. Get comfy. Create an ambient vibe to naturally transport you into a relaxed state. If you don't feel like you get the chance to, make time and make it something you look forward to! Focus on the routine habits that help you find elusive zen.

Massage

A technique not practiced enough among us is nighttime massage. Not only is it a beautiful way to relax, but a massage is also just a moment away from a good mood. A massage takes your mind from the past and the future and focuses on the present. Massages can be done in any form, from a professional method, with an acupressure mat, to a tennis or spike ball rolled along your back or feet. Massages activate your lymphatic system, which is a fantastic way to relieve tension from the day, loosen your body, and set a relaxing tone for a good night's sleep. We will touch on more techniques in the self-care ritual chapter.

The Beauty of Choice

An evening full of relaxation can include having a soak in the bath with Epsom salts, reading a book, practicing yoga, taking a tea to bed, having a glass of wine, watching a movie, socializing over dinner with friends, or even learning a new skill.

Evenings should be simple. Doing less and stressing less. This will ultimately help you to wake up feeling your best, setting yourself up to live a more beautiful life. Incorporating these few tips and practicing them daily will put you on the right path. You will feel a difference immediately. Setting up a routine lets you become the master of your life, and so you should be.

CHAPTER 3

MEDITATION AND MINDFULNESS

"Calm mind brings inner strength
and self-confidence, so that's very
important for good health."

—*Dalai Lama*

BE MINDFUL

When you are centered, you believe you can conquer anything. Transforming your state of mind will transform you, your body, and your being. After all, health is wealth, so why not create a sense of happiness within—in your mind—and without—in your body.

The effect of mindfulness is holistic. Mindful practices evoke a feeling of intention. They raise your vibration and help you live fully in the present moment. There is an interrelationship between the body and the mind. By practicing mindful activities, you will construct a beautiful life with positive influence and change.

Today, many people apply ancient traditions, such as meditation and mindful practices, to help battle stress, trauma, anxiety, and daily life. With such traditions can come surprisingly profound results. Starting small and increasing your practices will guide your body into a natural rhythm of creating space for mindfulness. The important thing to remember about mindfulness is that it is a skill. New skills require practice and familiarity.

Practicing meditation and mindfulness can easily become an essential part of your day. Meditation is a mindfulness practice, and just ten to fifteen minutes per day will deeply nurture your body and your inner self. To achieve a sense of mindfulness and introspection, you need to dig deep within yourself. Expand your worldview and master mental resilience to curate a sense of calm for your body, your mind, and your well-being. Like anything in life, when you take the time to train, you become great. When you learn to train your mind, you naturally and intuitively discover a world of greatness.

Mindfulness can also be heightened through external bodily practices. Being outdoors can be very meditative, and being in nature is truly grounding, which enhances that mind-body connection. Nature has an anti-inflammatory effect on the body. Mindful practices, like gardening, give a sense of purpose and offer physical enjoyment. All while getting some vitamin D, which can improve cognitive function and increase brain health. And, studies show that gardening is an incredibly therapeutic activity and can reduce depression and anxiety symptoms by easing stress and improving your mood—truly, the most inexpensive remedy!

There are many other ways to be outside and practice meditation all at the same time. Daily walks in nature, watching a sunrise or catching a sunset, picking flowers, walking in the grass, getting your toes in the sand, swimming, cycling, and watching the world simply run are all therapeutic, mindful practices. Allowing yourself to become anchored in connection with your mind and body in the present moment is vital to your well-being. Being in nature has a cathartic effect and can naturally elevate mood and energy levels. And the best part is that accessing the earth is free! We can all put our toes in the grass, our hands in the dirt, and our feet in the sand and the ocean. Whatever activity is uplifting and soothing for your mind and body should be what you continue to practice every day. Finding what works for you is the key to personal happiness.

WHY MEDITATION?

The mind and the body are so intertwined. You could argue they are inseparably one. It is important that we nourish the body, but it's equally important that we nourish the mind. Meditation helps to familiarize ourselves with feelings of stillness and contentment. Venturing beyond our usual routines, it intuitively forces us to luxuriate in the present moment. As we all know, time is precious, and the true control of life belongs to awareness, producing a heightened sensation of fullness. Being more mindful of where we focus our time and energy is essential in cultivating a beautiFUL(L) life.

Regardless of your present circumstances, I want to encourage you to have an open mind. Move past your doubts. Enhance your focus on your self-health. Create meditative space in your routine. There are limitless possibilities. Realize just how much your life improves when you have an open mind. It's amazing how fluid and effortless your life and everyday reality can be when your worldview shifts. Create the life you desire as if your life depends on it...because it does!

As this book unfolds, learn the beneficial enhancement you will receive when you assert your attention with intention. As they say, "Where attention goes, energy flows."

Vitality

Having a heightened sense of vitality comes with exuberant mental vigor. A person of great vitality is someone who practices being strong mentally and physically through practices like meditation. Research shows that the benefits of meditation include increased energy, mood, and quality sleep. All three of which aid clearer thinking for a stronger mentality and, therefore, vitality. Not only will meditation strengthen the inner you, but it will also strengthen the outer you too.

Intention

Consistency is key. Getting yourself to commit to a practice, a lifestyle, and a new you is challenging—let's not dismiss that—but what makes it easier to overcome the challenge is to be consistent. During times of questioning and non-believing, push through it. You will come out better on the other side and thank yourself a million times over for being intentional and committed. Wellness and peace of mind are about consistency. Staying consistent with yourself and your practice or routine will bring lasting results. Consistency is the main ingredient that holds it all together. Life doesn't ever get easier; you just get stronger. Showing up every day is a sense of achievement. The place where peace lives, even among the chaos, is when you commit to yourself intentionally and consistently. Meditation quiets the noise and grounds you in the present moment. Coming back day after day is where lasting change takes place.

Control

Being in control of your life is a beautiful thing. You are the controller of your time, feelings, actions, and so much more. We are all-powerful, and showing gratitude for ourselves and our potential is important. To master yourself, you must control yourself. In the new paradigm, the sense of control in life belongs to increased self-awareness. There is no special secret—it just has to be important enough to you to live a life full of opportunity and abundance.

Learning how to do so is a key role in meditation. Channeling your inner happiness, awareness, and thoughts is a way to discover who you truly are and what you need to manage to be who you want to be. Make it important enough to continue through any distraction or self-doubt. Recognize you feel better when you are consistent and move through life intentionally.

You can learn to control and leverage your stress, anxiety, and life responses through breathwork, which is a huge part of meditation. Breath is a life force. It's what makes you alive. It works by recalibrating your body's natural alignment. Controlling your breath is a great tool for controlling the mind. Therefore, if you can master breathwork, you can control yourself.

Presence

To achieve your highest sense of mindfulness, you must be present. Focusing on your present self and your surroundings instead of the past and the future will allow you to be aware of your thoughts and actions in a nonjudgmental manner. Being present and mindful is the core benefit of meditation and will allow you to communicate how you are thinking and feeling to both yourself and others.

Noticing the inseparable relationship between the body and mind will allow for enhanced well-being. If you are not aware of what your body needs, you cannot take care of it. This is why cultivating sensory awareness is critical. Thus, a distressed mental state can easily be converted into the biochemicals that create disease. The two go hand in hand through a mind-body connection. This is often why people with good mental health teach their bodies to age well. By living more presently, you will allow yourself to live in the essence of timelessness. Your awareness will become transcendent, and from that, you will feel a great sensation of fullness.

A MEDITATION GUIDE

While most people feel they need to go to a class to meditate, that is not true at all. The beautiful thing about meditation is that you can practice it almost anywhere. Anywhere that is calm and comfortable is a place where you can meditate. Find yourself a space where you can effectively clear your thoughts, and use that as a place to practice from daily.

Also, do not believe that meditation must be done in silence. If taking a walk, listening to music, or cooking your favorite meal helps you be mindful and calm, then do that! If it can clear your mind and let you reap the benefits of the practice, so be it.

You may be wondering how, exactly, to meditate. It is a very simple practice, and all you need is yourself and a quiet place to be able to do so. Meditation will allow you to get a fresh, unexpected perspective, whether you are a beginner or experienced. The best mind-body techniques to insert into living your beautiful life blueprint are listed below.

Set Achievable Goals

Start small. One to two minutes a day is enough to practice and get a feel for meditation. The best advice for meditation is to set achievable goals. Whether you are new to meditation or someone who has truly tried meditation and given up (like me), start small and realistic. Do it for one minute. Starting small is the answer to success. It reinforces the idea that you can do it. Just showing up for yourself is already a success! As you feel more comfortable and mindful, your practice will naturally get longer. Around fifteen minutes per day is an idyllic goal to aim for once you have mastered your meditation technique. Create a vibe—whether it be music, scent, or space. Then, make it something you look forward to.

Meditate First Thing Each Morning

Allow yourself a fresh, unexpected perspective. A daily practice of quiet allows us to become more present, more creative, and more open. Setting this intention will allow you to go about your day with a sense of gratitude, happiness, and mindfulness.

Check in with How You Are Feeling

Listen to your body and your mind to see what perspective you want to focus on. Each new practice will bring new emotions, and working on it day by day is a great way to grow. You will notice the more practiced you become at being present, the more intuitive you become.

Breathe Better

When you can, sit comfortably, count your breaths, and see how your stomach rises and falls through each passing breath. You may not be able to keep this up throughout the entire practice, as you may find your mind wanders, and that is okay. But, when you get the chance, focus on anchoring your mind and deliberate breathing, counting each inhale and exhale. There is power and connection from tuning in to your breath and body that stimulates enhanced awareness. These simple breathing techniques can energize your nervous system and calm your nerves. You will be amazed how quickly you begin to feel more alive.

Come Back When You Wander

Try not to stray with whatever arises in your mind, and stay on track throughout your practice, so you feel satisfied after. When, and if, you find your mind trailing off onto other thoughts, come back to your original focus so that you can wrap up on a positive, envigored path. The mind is our most precious resource, through which we experience every single moment of life. Do not beat yourself up if your mind wanders. Taking the time to sit and simply be still is looking after your mind, and there is no downside to that.

Turn Your Attention Inward

When your mind and heart are open, abundance will flow effortlessly and easily. Practicing meditation can become a part of your daily routine with a little extra effort. Turn your attention, quiet the mind, and soothe your senses. It's not about doing things correctly. It's about showing up and doing things that align with you and what feels real and authentic. The basic idea is to focus on that which makes you feel good and live well. Through interoceptive awareness, you can better develop the skills and emotional regulation to influence how you feel. This hidden sense of well-being, when attuned, will move you through the experience of living fully. After all, true beauty and health always shine from within.

HOW TO BE MINDFUL IN OTHER WAYS

There is an undeniable radiance from someone who is willing to grow, heal, and thrive. There are many other ways to be mindful. Self-development practices are a key part of developing a sense of mindfulness. While meditation is a great way to practice mindfulness daily, there are other methods that you might like to try each day. Your practices should involve enhancing a calm, strong mind while focusing more on the present moment.

Mindfulness is a basic human ability that involves a psychological process in which you bring your present self to the moment without judgment, which is what you learn through meditation and practicing gratitude. Suspending your judgment and unleashing natural curiosity in an overworked mind can help you approach a new and improved mentality, which will help you to be positive when being present.

Here are some things, other than meditation, that will help you practice mindfulness:

Self-Care Rituals

You may find that self-care rituals improve your mood and help channel your thoughts and body into a positive state to help with being in the moment. Creating a habit of pampering your body, mind, and spirit will feed you with good energy. We can face anything with grace and equanimity when we are centered. The simple act of taking care of yourself from the inside out can pay dividends.

Self-care allows a person to take control of their own mental, physical, and emotional state. It should be a daily practice to feel better. We all lead busy lives that sometimes stop us from putting ourselves first, but realizing we sometimes need more than we are giving is a misstep we all learn from. Taking a step back and noticing you need to love yourself first encourages integrating self-care rituals into your daily routine. Design the life you want. You are the architect of your life. Use your time wisely to create the space for self-care that you ultimately enjoy and look forward to while simultaneously enhancing your well-being. The effect is "wholistic."

While self-care may feel like a luxury (or even a selfish feeling), it is necessary to enhance your quality of life and those around you. Self-care means giving yourself permission to pause and putting yourself at the top of your to-do list. When you give yourself time and space to replenish your spirit, it allows you to serve others with your overflow of care and love. The relationship you have with yourself is more important than any other. Self-care is the wealth of your soul ("soul-care"), and the ultimate investment you can make is in supporting your health in mind, body, and spirit, and we know your mind is your strongest muscle!

Practicing self-care involves asking yourself what you need in the present moment and following through with it. Self-care rituals mean pressing into your mental routine as much as your physical routine—incorporating meditation, yoga, reading, walking, sleeping, and other activities that help physically and mentally. These are activities that help you forget everyday stresses and take a moment for yourself. They can also be more pampering, upgraded moments, such as an infrared sauna or steam session that serves a dual purpose—providing a physical detox as well as a mental one. If you don't have access to one, a quick cold rinse for the last thirty seconds of your shower is enough to reinvigorate your mind and awaken your senses. Adding one or more of these to your daily routine will help you feel a difference immediately. Life is precious. It's okay to pause and take time to be good to yourself.

Caring for yourself is an act of self-love and nurturing. It helps increase your capacity for impact and progresses your new ways of living beautiful. Life is all about choices. Who makes those choices? You! Mindfulness paves the way for a kinder world, one that you can greatly impact.

Beautiful Escape

Our living space is truly our personal sanctuary. Or at least it should be! Make it a beautiful space to live. As a place where you often escape to or find comfort in after the stressors of daily life, your home needs to evoke a serene atmosphere to help you restore and rejuvenate.

Sometimes, all you need to reset your wellness routine is an upgrade to your space. Create a relaxed feel that instantly warms your soul. Nature provides us with so many mood-boosting endorphins. Bring nature indoors with some natural elements, whether it be natural light, fresh-cut flowers, accessorized bowls of fruit, or a beautiful carafe with freshly sliced citrus. You deserve a space that refreshes your senses and instantly feels like a welcome home.

Set the tone of your space that emulates you. Hang inspiring artwork. Invest in rousing and decorative table books. Create positive nostalgia through your personal aesthetic and with photos of your favorite memories.

Make your self-care (or living beautiful) a priority and your prescription for living well. Studies show that improving your space helps to nurture your creativity and thoughts, engaging your mind in newfound and meaningful ways. It's the small things that can make the biggest difference in your space. Why not enjoy it?

Current Mood: Calm

Now, more than ever, embracing joy and making time for the things that make you truly happy—from quiet moments of reflection and pampering to anything that nourishes your soul—is important. Simply upgrade your space. When you spend more time at home, your surroundings must reflect a sense of calm and comfort.

Create an escape at home. Awaken your senses. Use refreshing scents and enhancements to reinvigorate your space, enhance your mood, and give you a new, fresh, and sound perspective. Neutral tones in natural fibers create a sense of serenity and light in your living space by adding calming scent and comforting decor. Invest in blankets and linens that bring solace and relaxation throughout. Diffuse scent in your home or workspace. Light candles, burn sage, play tranquil music. Give your body what it craves. Relax and recharge with mindless music that makes you feel good yet does not make you think, eliciting a mindless escape. Creating this space sets the tone for your spirit and how you can manage your day and your everyday stressors.

Improving Your Sleeping Pattern

Sleep is a vital component of our lives, a necessary component of our health, well-being, and happiness. Getting enough sleep works wonders in many ways. It can help reduce stress, increase concentration, boost productivity, maximize athletic performance, and improve immunity. Not to mention, it can also have a profound effect on your appearance. Sleep is medicine. Getting enough sleep is easier said than done. So, each one of us needs to sacrifice things to tune into relaxation and sleep.

Investing in rest means cutting out caffeine and giving up your phone, a chore, or your favorite TV show to get in the right mindset to sleep. Prioritizing sleep is an act of self-love, and should be seen as a necessity over other not-so-important things.

The best way to get more sleep is by simply going to sleep earlier and waking up earlier. This goes back to making a new life-style—a new routine and schedule to balance your work and personal life.

Balance in your routine will lead to having more freedom with your schedule. It will allow you to prioritize things you may not necessarily be prioritizing currently, like sleep. Switching off your phone, leaving work on time, and small life changes can help you get into bed earlier and get to sleep before your usual time.

Build a bedtime routine and a consistent sleep schedule, waking up as close to the same time each day. Seven to eight hours of sleep is enough for most people to function at their best level. An improved sleeping pattern will manage stress both mentally and physically to nurture your body from the outside in. Be grateful for closing your eyes and resting your mind and body.

Eating Your Medicine

Remember, the benefit of getting healthier is to maximize what your body can do for you. Nourishing your body with the right nutrients is not a mystical concept. In fact, eating mind-fully can help you in several ways. It can aid better digestion, regulate appetite, and make us appreciate and be grateful for the food we eat.

Tuning into what we eat can help us make better life choices, not just better diet choices. Foods that boost your immune system and nutrients that can nourish your nervous system are what you need to consume if you want to eat mindfully. See food as your medicine. All food contains phytonutrients, which are chemicals made up of minerals, vitamins, or nutrients. They are special proteins that interact with your natural body's science and speak to your genes. When you think of food, think color. Fill your diet with vegetables and goodness.

Colorful foods can transform your health as well as your life. What we choose to put into our bodies significantly affects everything from our mood to our cognitive function. Food is medicine, and the right foods care for your body as much as exercise, sleep, and self-care do. Like all other aspects that improve your mind, body, and soul, you should follow what your mind and body want to eat. Eating should be a pleasure and not something done absentmindedly. Focus on what you want and should eat, and follow your gut. Eating right does not mean only eating healthy foods. If you want a slice of cake or a cocktail, then have it. But know when and how to limit processed and sugary foods. Eating them all the time is not healthy, but occasionally treating yourself will help your mind and body stay on track. What your body needs is balance. Focus on mindful eating while knowing what works best for your body. When it comes to mindful eating, it is really about mindful living and living fully!

Your pantry should be full of good and nutritious food to eat right. Find healthy foods that work for you—foods that you will enjoy consuming on a daily basis to stay on track.

Immune-boosting recipes include nutritious, balanced foods that are essential to consume every day. These foods contain good fats and healthy calories, which can be found in foods like nuts, dark leafy greens, fatty fish, and whole grains. These foods are good for your gut, heart, and nervous system, aiding good digestion and energy. They will make you feel your best, stay on track, and feel mindful and nourished, which is exactly what you need.

Think of food as a practice and a way to improve the life and diet choices you make. Live by the mantra "Mind. Body. Medicine."

Later in the book, you will find more on the best-balanced foods, recipe enhancements, supplements, and more, so stay tuned if you are interested in how to eat your medicine and use your pantry as your pharmacy.

Being Beautiful

Being the best version of yourself, putting yourself first, giving your body what it needs, and tuning into your feelings will undoubtedly improve your mental health. Ensuring your mental health is balanced is key in taking the next step to living beautiful. Not every day is actually the best day ever. Life is not that simple. But each day collectively makes up our weeks, which make up our years, which make up our lives. If you work on your mental health and give your mind, body, and soul what it needs, you are making a choice to live your best life that is uniquely you. Because who we are in a lifetime is a collection of who we are each day.

Being kind to yourself and learning to practice mindfulness every day, even in small doses, will make living the best version of yourself easier. Channeling your inner feelings and expressing them as best you can will help you understand yourself better. Acknowledging and expressing your feelings is the step you need towards living a beautiful life.

Being beautiful is not about physical appearance, nor should it be about wanting others to think you are beautiful. Before you wish for others to appreciate you, you should wish to appreciate yourself.

Physical appearance does not reflect what is on the inside. A day where you feel you are physically looking your best may be a day when you are mentally not feeling your best. What is on the outside is not a true representation of what is on the inside. Changing your perspective on life and working on what you want to improve in your life comes from improving what is on the inside.

Happiness is letting go of what you think your life is supposed to look like and celebrating it for everything that it is. Being beautiful comes from within. Once you have mastered that, living beautiful will soon follow.

CHAPTER 4

TRACK YOUR HABITS

"If I cannot do great things, I can do small things in a great way."

—Martin Luther King Jr.

STAY ON TRACK

The beautiful thing about your life is that you are in charge of your time. The only one who can control how your day goes is you. Like everyone, you have commitments, but ultimately, you control your hours, minutes, and seconds.

It is never too late to regenerate your life. Mind and body dynamics are like muscle memory; you will never lose your rhythm and technique once you establish it. Having control of your time means that your every movement is chosen by you, so prioritize your habits and rituals.

If you want to spend your time wisely, tracking your habits is the best thing to introduce into your life. Writing down your habits and what you've achieved every day will give you a sense of accomplishment.

Tracking your habits, from small to big steps, can help you feel in control of your destiny. It helps you be and become more practical. A balanced lifestyle brings your mind, body, and spirit into unity. From new and improved habits, you will feel more fulfillment in every area of your life.

Your inner self knows better than anyone and anything how your life is meant to go. So, tracking your daily movements, tasks, and more will help lead you along the right path and help you stay on track.

To find what works best for you, start by tracking one health habit a day.

Habit tracking can help you make healthy habits a way of life if you struggle with prioritizing yourself and making healthy choices. Stress and bad habits greatly contribute to poor health. Poor habits can negatively impact your body long-term. One of the best things you can do for yourself is to always care for your body and make it your prerogative. Put your self-care on a higher priority list. Creating habits is truly an art. But making small changes is a great way to cultivate the seeds of good habits. This will vastly improve your quality of life, which your body will thank you for.

For example, if you aren't giving yourself enough water during the day or you are lacking sleep, tracking this will help you recognize that. Noticing what you are lacking will help you improve.

Getting enough movement, water, sleep, and balanced food will soon become easier with habit tracking. There are countless tools that make it easy and nearly effortless to track your health habits, such as fitness apps, journals, and wearable devices. Start today. Develop a growth mindset. Track your food, your exercise, your steps (even if it is walking to and from work), your water intake, and how much quality sleep you get. Tomorrow, you will see patterns. The next day, you will notice even more of a pattern. Not only will this give you a sense of accomplishment, but you will naturally feel more in control of your life. This may be all the momentum you need to inspire better habits.

After a day or two, you will immediately spot your unhealthy habits and want to throw them out the window. Good. This will help you develop a strategy of small things you can do today to start feeling better. You will soon learn and want to make healthier food options, swap carbonated energy for water, turn your phone off earlier, and get more sleep. Even the smallest amount of restorative habits can influence enhanced well-being.

WHAT EXACTLY SHOULD YOU TRACK?

High on the list is the importance of health and prioritizing self-care. Daily movement, health habits, and chore checklists are the best things to start with when it comes to tracking your habits. These are the three activities that make up most of your day—the factors in your life you may want to change and improve upon. They are the most important parts of your life to focus on in order to live beautiful.

Tracking small things, such as your water intake, restful sleeping hours, meditative time, and when you eat, walk, exercise, or complete a task are things you can attain and check off throughout the day. Completing one of your daily habits allows you to move on to the next one. Being able to see what comes next— what you have prioritized—will allow you to get through each activity. Tracking is motivating.

For the greatest impact on your well-being, you should begin your habit tracking with two things:

Daily Movement

Movement every day is healthy. Movement allows us to express ourselves, our mentality, and our physicality. Whether you like to walk, run, do yoga, stretch, or play a sport, getting in daily exercise is imperative for a healthy mind and body.

A huge priority in life is to keep yourself moving. Movement is therapy. Exercise and movement allow you to give time to yourself, tune into your thoughts, and energize your body. It is invigorating, and movement plays an important role in a balanced lifestyle.

Without movement, a sense of un-accomplishment may encourage you to slack off. Failing to add movement into your day may decrease your motivation, as well as your routine and everything you have worked hard for in striving to live beautiful.

If you don't move enough, then make it a priority. Starting small will help motivate you, influencing greater productivity and performance. The habit of tracking your daily movement can be leveraged to accomplish and motivate you to do it again the next day.

Right now, if you are a person who doesn't get much physical activity due to your job (i.e., an office job which requires you to be at a desk all day), think of ways you can add more movement and exercise to your day. For example, you can try an alternative way to get to work that involves more walking or cycling. Or, if you can dedicate certain days to exercise classes during lunchtime or after work, then go for it. Finding ways to stay active can be mood boosting with minimal to zero cost or equipment needed.

Physical fitness is intimately linked to general well-being. Exercise has a holistic effect that will make you feel more balanced and more centered. Aim for at least thirty minutes of physical activity every day and create a modified weekday fitness schedule that works for you.

Hydration

An important health habit to begin is getting enough water. H_2O is your best friend, and your body needs water more than anything else in life. Water is essential for life, but drinking enough of it can also be one of the easiest things we neglect. All live beings—humans, animals, and plants—need water to survive. Hydrating is something you should add to your daily schedule, and remind yourself to drink throughout the day.

Drinking six cups of water every day and choosing herbal teas over other drinks is a great place to start. Green tea is especially good with powerful antioxidants, which flush your system, making you feel less sluggish and more energized. Or, to jazz up your water, you could try adding lemon, cucumber, lime, mint, basil, grapefruit, sage, rosemary, or any combination of them. Making it tasty and refreshing helps ensure you enjoy every sip while balancing your body's hydration.

Why begin with water? Dehydration leads to high cortisol levels, the stress hormone, which leads to high stress. High stress is one of the most detrimental issues for your health. It can take its toll on your mind, body, and soul. Nobody should wish stress upon themselves. The expression "you bloom where you are planted" is a reminder you can grow and thrive if you take care of yourself. Like plants, we all need water to flourish. Therefore, a small habit like drinking enough water will decrease stress, hydrate you, aid digestion and detoxification, and so much more—the list could go on forever.

Intermittent Fasting

Once you've mastered the movement and hydration habits, you can look for new habits to adopt. One habit you could practice is intermittent fasting one day a week. It is good for your gut, well-being, and health, and it is easy to track. After writing down the results and realizing how good it makes you feel, you will find the encouragement and motivation to continue.

Perhaps you have heard of intermittent fasting. If you have not, it is a fasting technique that enhances cellular repair and reduces inflammation. Fasting one day a week for a minimum of twelve hours is enough to see amazing results. It is a great addition to a healthier lifestyle and has an abundance of health benefits. Don't worry; we will cover it in more detail later.

Making small habits will inspire you to create more healthy habits when you notice how good it makes you feel. Once you master and manage to maintain these healthy habits, try adding more as the motivation comes to you. You will soon be tracking all that makes you happy and wish to improve upon.

WHERE AND HOW TO TRACK YOUR HABITS

Tracking your habits is best done manually. Strip back to basics to find out what method will work best. Everyone is different, so keep trying until you find the method that works best for you. Pen and paper methods, such as journals, notepads, vision boards, or a simple whiteboard, are easily available. You can begin straight away.

Having a habit schedule will allow you to keep track of your time as well as your habits; every hour, you can check in on your schedule and see what habit is next to accomplish.

Alternatively, you can write notes or make tables and charts to track each activity/task/accomplishment you have achieved. Make time for noting your habits the night before or the morning of so that you know what you need and want to accomplish each day. Over time, these habits become instinctual. Every day can be different or the same; you are the controller of your time and destiny, so long as you are keeping balance and creating healthy habits.

If the traditional pen and paper methods do not work for you, try using technology. Apps and computer software are other ways you can keep track of your daily habits. There are numerous phone apps for tracking your habits, such as Headspace, Calm, Oura, Insight Tracker, and Fitbit. These work just like to-do lists and charts and are easily accessible from your phone. Some may find using an app easier and more motivating as it can offer encouragement and reminders throughout the day.

Whatever tracking method works best for you, stick to it. It is the best way to stay motivated and keep up the routine of tracking your habits. Staying on track is key for building and maintaining a beautiful life.

WHY YOU SHOULD TRACK YOUR HABITS

Habit tracking motivates us to move forward and improve, which is very satisfying. Embrace the power of routine. Routines are key to optimal health and wellness. They help to enhance your life; they create regularity and sustainability. This impacts everything from mental health to digestive health, sleep, mood, energy levels, and more. If you're ready to get into a new routine, try tracking your habits this week, and notice how you feel.

A major benefit you can gain from tracking your habits is that you begin to consciously use your intuition; you pay closer attention to your body. This will benefit your health and well-being in the long run.

Your choices result in what path you take in life. What you do today can affect the quality of your health thirty or forty years from now. Tracking your habits allows you to control your destiny. If you make meaningful actions, live a meaningful life, and choose to invest your time, it means you will be successful in living beautiful. We each have a potential we are destined for, and fulfilling that is the ultimate meaning of controlling your own destiny.

Tracking your habits also allows you to be honest with yourself. Some of us go about our days thinking we've accomplished enough. Once you write down your habits and look back, you may realize you aren't doing as much as you thought, and you can do more.

Tracking your habits quantifies your actions, holds you accountable, and helps you decide whether you're making progress or not. If you find you are, then great. If you are not, then you can decide to change course and improve. We can only define our habits and what works for us with trial and error. There can be no right without any wrongs. Failure does not define weakness; it encourages us to be better.

WHO SHOULD TRACK YOUR HABITS?

Only you can track your habits. Only you can improve your quality of life, health, and well-being. You are the master of your time. It is easy for others to interfere with your schedule, which can derail your self-focus and commitments. Set boundaries, unlearn bad habits, and learn to be in control. Implement healthy habits in moderation, and do what feels authentic to you. After all, it is you and only you who can implement change and better yourself.

Be in charge of your own time in order to focus on doing things that bring you happiness and make you feel alive.

Tracking your habits is a task only you can do in order to be true to yourself. Denying yourself the space to moderate your time and your schedule will only hold you back from making healthier habits and life choices, so learn to liberally allocate your time when it comes to habit tracking.

Be truthful with yourself. You wouldn't put trust in another person who lies, so why would you put trust in yourself if you are dishonest. Honesty is the best policy, and being truthful with yourself will better your mind, soul, and habits.

If you're a master at making a habit and sticking to it, then that's fantastic. That is the exact attitude you need for success. However, if you are someone who easily falls out of a habit and needs some encouragement to stay on track, you are not alone. There is a reason why New Year's resolutions typically have a short shelf life. Tracking your habits can help you to sustain an "I can" attitude that often acts as the catalyst needed to encourage and motivate you. Keep these guidelines in mind if your habits break down:

Perfection Is Not Possible

Somewhere along the line, all of us break habits. This may be down to lack of motivation, or for those who are good at keeping habits, an emergency may pop up, which will break your streak. Don't panic; you can get it back.

Never Miss Twice

If you miss it one day, do everything you can to not miss it the next. Missing one scheduled workout or self-care session is okay, but missing out twice in a row makes it easier for you to fall out of the habit. Tell yourself that a day off is a way to regenerate. There is no need to lose track of a habit twice. Missing once is an accident. Missing twice is the start of a new habit.

Make Them Irresistible

Habits should not be an onerous or burdensome chore. Make them enticing—a ritual and daily regime you look forward to. Keep it practical to your everyday demands, but carve out that time for yourself, and make it so good you won't want to break the habit. Habits do not need to be restrictive. Strive to add one positive habit per week. It could be as basic as drinking more water by simply creating a beverage station in the comfort of your room or kitchen, using your favorite carafe to elevate your experience and more frequently hydrate. Another option is taking a meditative moment outside in the fresh air to yourself. It could also be getting to bed earlier by enriching and creating your evening wind-down routine—whether that be playing soothing music while taking a bath, diffusing luxurious, calming oil blends in your room, or indulging in a relaxing skin care regimen.

Refresh Your Routine

Small habits form success. No habits work unless you do. Your lifestyle is the sum of your habits. Adopt healthier habits by starting small. "Make it easy" is how James Clear, author of *Atomic Habits*, puts it. Do them daily. Prioritize yourself the moment you wake up each day with an intention to create and implement one health-enhancing exercise into your routine that is authentically you. It can be as simple as picking a time of day, turning off notifications on your phone, or creating a nonnegotiable wind-down routine.

Pair Your Habits

Create simple and mindless routines of good habits. It can be as simple as drinking your water while you go on a walk. Meditating while you do breathwork. Cooking while you listen to a podcast or audiobook that makes you feel good. The act of creating a routine that is sustainable and enjoyable is the main ingredient in building a repeatable and achievable routine of life-enhancing habits.

Tracking habits can boost your ability to form and sustain a healthy lifestyle. It allows you to become aware of your habits first, and then it helps you assess which you want to maintain and which you want to improve on. Without tracking your daily habits yourself, you may never realize what you need to improve on or what you are doing well with. There is a connection between achieving a better routine and increased health. Recognizing your achievements, successes, and failures is an important tool to live beautiful, and is made easier by tracking your own habits.

Your daily habits set the stage for your life, and fine-tuning behavioral changes is important for bettering yourself and recognizing your strengths, which many of us need to do more. We can be more productive when we prioritize our well-being. Set yourself up for success. The only person you should strive to be better than is who you were yesterday.

Living beautiful is possible, and you are the only person who can make it happen, so why not start tracking your habits to create a healthier life now?

CHAPTER 5

INVEST IN YOURSELF

"My mission in life is not merely to survive, but to thrive."

—Maya Angelou

TAKE A MOMENT

Expressing your best self means taking care of the most important component: you! Before you conquer the day, get centered wherever you are with whatever makes you feel your best, whether that be elevated moments of self-care or laid-back, simple, feel-good moments. Wellness is a state of mind. Set yourself up for a Zen start to your day by developing simple strategies to best treat your mind, body, and soul. Find your sweet spot. Once you understand yourself, you can live beauti-FULLY and become your healthiest self, inside and out. You have every right to a beautiful life.

Take a Breath

Enjoy Nature

Eat Whole Foods

Stay Hydrated

Listen to Good Music

Break a Sweat

Meditate

Embrace Solitude

Get Good Rest

Keep Going

NATURAL HABITAT

Getting outside has been incredibly healing in my wellness journey. There is something cathartic about being in nature. Breathing in the fresh air and listening to nature's soundscape can have a significant impact on your brain, mood, physiology, and overall well-being. As seasons change, take advantage of the milder weather by spending some time outside with a new book, trying your hand at gardening, or just enjoying some quiet time to walk or dine outside. It is a no-cost therapy that can nourish your psyche and naturally calm your nervous system. Don't underestimate the happiness effect of being outdoors. It is a no-cost remedy to nurture your soul.

YOUR MIND AND BODY BY YOUR DESIGN

We will all agree that a little escape is needed right now. Now, more than ever, we are aware that life is ours to appreciate, whether it's through a feel-good playlist, a new book, or the people we surround ourselves with. The self-care rituals we incorporate into our daily routines affect our mental health and overall well-being. Surrounding yourself with positive influences and rituals that make you happy and act as a form of escapism matter most for our mental health. Taking time to slow down and renew ourselves is imperative. Practicing self-care is important in tough times and at all times.

Although we are all students of our own lives, through learning about ourselves every day, we are also the architects of our lives. You are the project leader for your health, well-being, and happiness. Being present will help you become an accomplished creator of your own destiny.

As we become more in tune with our bodies, we acknowledge how to orchestrate and guide our behavior, uniting body and mind—living a truly beautiful life. Your life is yours to relish. Put into practice what radiates your true self.

CURRENT MOOD: CALM

When spending more time at home, it's important that your surroundings reflect a sense of calm and comfort. CREATE YOUR CALM. Cultivate your own sense of space with style and design elements that inspire you, and make you feel relaxed, reinvigorated, or pampered. As long as your space cultivates the positive mood you want to foster, you cannot go wrong.

If you want to create a calming atmosphere, start by scenting your space with natural aromatherapeutic blends. It is so easy to find diffusers these days for aromatherapy. You can use scent to lift your mood and awaken your senses with white florals, sparkling citrus, and fresh green accords, leaving you feeling energized and centered. This is a perfect addition to your home office or, even better, your bedroom to prompt your wind-down routine.

Learn to simplify your space and elevate the ordinary. Create a light and airy space that is simply for you. See it as a moment to be still, even if it is a place of calm you use for five minutes a day.

Be mindful and purposeful about creating warmth, comfort, and quiet moments of reflection. Swap candles for artificial light, keep a cozy throw for ultimate comfort when you take that time to meditate, journal, or simply reflect. Be in the present, and let your surroundings nurse you. There is a reason why they say "There is no place like home."

THE VALUE OF INWARD FOCUS

Now that you've put meditation, mindfulness, habit tracking, better nourishment, and more into practice, it's time to invest in yourself. Time to enrich your life for the long haul. Time to incorporate all of these practices into your life and make time for them. If you've mastered those skills and habits, you have even more power to focus on yourself.

We all need to—and deserve to—be selfish at times. You need to self-prioritize and practice self-compassion if you want to be truly selfless. The path to selflessness requires an obligatory commitment to take care of yourself. There is a reason why they say "You cannot pour from an empty cup." Focus on making healthy life choices and treating your body right. Taking the time to invest in yourself helps you practice self-compassion, self-love, self-care, self-esteem, self-respect, and self-management. To connect to the highest version of yourself, you have to look inside. Selfishness will help you appreciate yourself, better yourself, and focus on yourself. This self-compassion will reveal the naturally compassionate, loving, caring person you are. Challenge yourself to identify your gifts and talents. The investment is worth it.

The poet Rumi said it this way: "Let the beauty of what you love be what you do." We must focus inward, re-evaluate ourselves, and find what truly motivates us to live fully. Get clear on your purpose, set an intention, and focus on those habits that allow you to show up as the best version of yourself.

SELF-CARE AND SELF-LOVE: THE FOUNDATION

In times of difficulty, it's more important than ever to take a moment to show a little kindness to the person who matters most in your life: yourself. Your body needs self-care rituals for your mental and emotional well-being. Practical acts of self-care are so important for good physical and mental health. Once you start practicing new habits and self-care practices, they soon become a fluid part of your daily routine. According to psychology reports, it takes twenty-one days to create a new habit. Let this habit formation be a mental reset. After a few weeks of having a new daily routine, it will unconsciously feel like an inherent and natural part of your life, and you will be surprised to see how much your body craves it!

Remember, you are the architect of your life and the only one with the vision board. It is the little things you do daily that allow you to become the architect of your destiny. Live as though it is your career. Think of it this way: you have a solo project, and it is you and only you who can complete that project from start to finish; you are the designer of that project—the only person who can determine its results. Think of your journey to living beautiful the same way. You can choose to take care of yourself.

It is you who chooses whether or not you want to improve your habits, better yourself as a person, and practice new habits in order to live a healthier and happier life. It is you who has the power to change your life, and understanding that is essential in creating positive change. It is you who needs to put into practice daily rituals to successfully sustain and better your life.

Simple strategies like sleep, exercise, meditation, food, hydration, "me moments," and digital free time are great ways to bring out your inner happiness, focus on what your body needs, and transform your state of mind. Transforming your mind will quickly put you in the right mindset to transform whatever you wish. Whether you want to improve your body, your food habits, your work, or your self-care routine, putting your mind in the right place and incorporating these steps into your everyday life will help with that. Even if it is only one thing. Have a high appreciation for the simple experiences and pleasures of life.

In these moments of self-care, be enraptured by the beauty of life. Whether through watching a sunset, meditating at sunrise, or losing yourself in a book, take your time to disconnect from life and connect to nature. Feel and nurture the beauty of the world in every moment that you can. You are the content creator of your life. What you take in, you hold with you. This internal energy will ground you and be exuded to others around you. When we can establish habits, practices, and routines of self-love, we will find ourselves to be more authentic and honest. We will tend to enforce healthy boundaries in relationships, and we will be more grateful and compassionate. Not only will this make you more beautiful and loving, but how we make ourselves feel extends to how we make others feel.

GOOD NIGHT, SLEEP TIGHT

Your emotional and mental health are intimately related to the quality of your sleep, and how you rest your body and mind. Look at sleep as your best investment. The beneficial enhancements you will receive in getting good quality sleep are profound. Consider it the greatest insurance policy for your health that comes at no cost. While we sleep, we allow for a reset and recharge, improving how we function mentally, physically, and cognitively. However, not all rest is good rest. The quality of your sleep influences the quality of your life. Today, there are many things you can do to facilitate a better night's sleep—from morning routines to wind-down rituals—and, as a result, you will discover a healing power, naturally elevated energy levels, increased immune health, and better skin. Studies show that improving your sleep means improving your immune system, mental clarity, creativity, memory, and more.

There is a real connection between sleep and how we heal our bodies. When you allow your body and mind to rest deeply, you experience a new quality of authenticity and self-care. Take time to uncover restorative sleep rituals. Better sleep is the cornerstone to better health. Prepare your body and mind for a good quality night's sleep. As the sun begins to set, your body's natural circadian rhythm adjusts for winding down. Find time to steep a balancing cup of tea, slip into something cozy, or indulge yourself with a restorative skin care routine to relax your body and mind. Winding down can be effortlessly facilitated by the environment you create. Allow for a transcendental and nocturnal space. Make it peaceful by reducing clutter, keeping it at a cool temperature, and minimizing artificial light. Illuminate your room with candles and diffuse calming scented oils. The environment you create can set the tone for your body to enter a more relaxed state. A soothing bedtime routine is a critical part of your ability to fall asleep. It's not always as easy as switching our minds off like our smartphones. Adding even one of these simple practices can create a space of calm as you prepare your body for rest.

My clean-sleep prescription is filling my diffuser with a mix of lavender and eucalyptus oil, hiding my cell phone at least an hour before bed, and sipping something calming with a book in hand. It's almost foolproof.

JOURNAL: LET IT ALL OUT

We spoke about journaling earlier, but the subject is worth revisiting. Simply put pen to paper, and use this time as a healthy way to open up and authentically express yourself. At the beginning or end of each day, sit down with your thoughts. Use this as a time to review what you did, what you thought, and what could be improved in your day. The way you write does not need to follow any certain structure. It's your own private place to discuss and create whatever you want to express about your current feelings and musing thoughts. Let the words and ideas flow freely. Don't worry about spelling mistakes or what other people might think.

It doesn't matter when or how you journal. The point is to establish a mindfulness routine that is simple and feels right. Notice what contributes to your happiness and what detracts from it. Writing your thoughts keeps you in the present moment and can pointedly define your sense of awareness. Embrace the impermanence, and become present with your thoughts.

Cultivate a heightened sense of awareness and serenity by anchoring yourself in the present moment. In the future, it will be remarkable to look back on your thoughts and see how you've grown and persevered through difficult thoughts or relished in happy times.

Look at your writing time as personal relaxation time. It's a time when you can de-stress and wind down. Write in a place that's relaxing and soothing, maybe with a cup of coffee or tea. Look forward to this time and know that you're doing something great for your mind and body.

Journaling is a great way to check in with yourself, engage your focus, and practice self-awareness. Take time out of your day to create intentions, build habits, and understand the best version of yourself with the journal prompts below:

- grateful

- intention

- feel

- movement

- learn

- self-care

- get done

- inspiration

- send love

FEEL VIBRANT AND ELEVATE YOUR LIFE

I want to convince you that you are much more than your limited body, spirit, and personality. The most meaningful thing you can live for is to reach your full potential.

When you feel better, you will learn to live more. You will understand that feeling elevated in your health, motivation, kindness, self-care, and daily practices will help you live a better version of yourself. Remodeling yourself isn't necessarily changing you as a person. Instead, it is allowing yourself to invest in your well-being, nourishment, movement, and self-love.

Learn to love yourself and what you are doing to successfully transform your body, life, and state of mind. You are so much more powerful than you might think. Your body is a temple; your mind is as wide, strong, and powerful as you make it. Reinforcing your awareness to create the life you want is up to you. Focusing your power, energy, and control on the way you want your life to unfold comes with practice and patience.

As humans, we can face anything with grace, solace, and equanimity when we are centered. This goes back to focusing on your mind before your body. When the mind is in the right place, the rest of your life can also be. Your happiness is inside you; it just takes practice to bring it out.

FEEL BEAUTIFUL

It is important to understand that while being fit does not define one's worth, the act of caring for your body is an investment in yourself. Finding a good balance of exercise that works for you and your body's needs without overdoing it is key.

In addition to your mental state, it is also essential to take good care of your physical state. Although appearance isn't everything, it does contribute to how you feel. Feeling like you look good helps with confidence and motivation, and it contributes to a healthier mindset.

Looking after your body begins in your gut. As mentioned earlier, hydration is of the utmost importance, and it is key for your gut health. Flushing away toxins with plenty of water throughout the day will keep your internal organs hydrated. If you find it difficult to drink water because of a lack of taste, remember you can add fruits or herbs to your water to improve the taste and add health benefits. A few slices of lemon in your water can increase detoxification and alkalinity, which will help your gut feel better, and help you feel more energized. A healthy gut is good for sustaining energy levels.

A healthier gut helps build a strong immune system, which helps stave off illnesses. Luckily, there are numerous ways to improve your immune system: from getting enough sleep to having a healthy diet. The beautiful lifestyle choices you can make will help your body to heal, your immune system to strengthen, your mind to stay on track, and you to feel beautiful. We will discuss in later chapters the importance of a healthy gut and its impact on your muscles, energy stores, and immune response.

BOUNDARIES: THE BEAUTY OF CHOICE

Epictetus, a Greek Stoic philosopher said, "You are not your body and hairstyle, but your capacity for choosing well. If your choices are beautiful, so too will you be." You can be the change in your world. It is you who can make a real difference in creating new habits and diminishing old ones. If you turn up every day and take a little time to practice well-being, nutrition, movement, and self-care, that is an accomplishment that will upgrade your life. Wellness is about the tiny moments when you show up and give yourself the love that sustains and supports you.

Just remember: Love yourself first. Invest in yourself first. Chase your dreams. Protect your peace. Make mistakes and learn from them. Life is all about choices. Choosing to live more beautiful, productively, and peacefully leads to a new generation of kind, compassionate, and openhearted human beings. Believe in yourself. Be intentional about the thoughts you focus on. Be intentional about what you consume. By starting on this new path and making a concerted effort towards your intellectual self-care, you will soon see others lead with you to better their lives.

CHAPTER 6

FOOD FOR THOUGHT

*"But the real secret to lifelong good
health is actually the opposite: Let
your body take care of you."*
—Deepak Chopra

EAT BEAUTIFUL

Food impacts our lives in a myriad of ways. Your diet is not only what you eat, it's also what you watch, what you listen to, what you read, and even the people you surround yourself with. Be mindful of the things you are putting into your body emotionally, physically, and spiritually. All of these little things add up.

Diet comes from the Greek word *dieta* which means "way of life." Being presently mindful of what you are enjoying and feeding your body should be the ultimate focus. Dieting is a thing of the past. Consumption should be a mindful practice while offering you inner peace and freedom from your food choices. Strive to eat mindfully with real, whole foods and declare a new meaning for diet: discover, influence, enhance, transform.

Your internal environment is influenced by your mind. How you define *diet* matters. Being mindful of the things you are consuming in every part of life will help you achieve optimal wellness. There is a need for significant habit formation in these areas, and the benefits you will receive are significant.

NOURISH TODAY, TRANSFORM TOMORROW

Proper nutrition is the key to physical, emotional, and even spiritual health. Food is an experience of life, and we should enjoy ourselves through nutritious foods, as well as our favorite foods. It is our nourishment and is the major driver in how we look, how we feel, and how we perform. Your internal health boosts your outer radiance. There is a healing power in nutrition. Food controls our body's ability to defend itself in a multitude of ways. What we choose to put into our bodies affects not only our mood but our cognitive function. Small changes—when done with consistency—create lasting change in every way our body functions.

The work you put into your health is profound and powerful. What you perpetuate through nourishment can aid in attaining the highest quality of life. At the end of the day, pleasure must be the main ingredient. You need to live a happy life, which is achieved by consuming pleasurable things.

I am inviting you to shift your perspective and view cooking and eating food as an opportunity to experiment with new flavors. Make life more colorful, exciting, and wholesome in your kitchen. Incorporate these dietary shifts to achieve long-term wellness and lead a beautiful life in which all of the right ingredients come together.

NATURAL NURTURING

Nurturing your body with the utmost care—from the inside out—is one of the most important aspects of maintaining a healthy lifestyle. What most people do not realize is that in order to start feeling better, taking care of your insides is the first step.

Food Is Medicine

The saying goes, "An ounce of prevention is worth a pound of cure." Try to get your nutrition from food, if possible. Choosing the right foods will help you become an early champion of prevention, all while enhancing your body's function and optimizing your overall health. Combat health issues with intuitive eating. Eat creatively and artistically to improve your life and your health. Step out of your comfort zone, and add color to your world with food.

Ayurveda

A pseudoscientific practice that stems from deep within Indian culture, Ayurveda is a medicine-based diet founded over three thousand years ago to support mindfulness. The key reason for introducing an element of Ayurveda into your life is to promote balance. You can influence every aspect of your health right now through your immune system and by adding balance to the way you live life. Those influences can be dietary, stress reduction, exercise related, and even the quality of your relationships. In addition to the supporting psychological effects, incorporating this mindset of Ayurveda can supply your body with nutritional balance.

The Basics

In today's ever-changing, chaotic world, sometimes simple is better. Going back to basics with your diet can prove to be worthwhile and very beneficial. Focus on living healthier. Eliminating superficial foods and inflammatory ingredients from your diet promotes good health. As proven by evolution, our bodies were designed to eat wholesome and natural foods. Before the age of toxic chemicals found in foods, the human body was less susceptible to diseases, both self-causing and hereditary. Food is an enormous pathway to health and healing.

Fruits

A wholesome, natural, and historic healing food, fruits have adaptogenic and antiaging properties. They have been around for millions of years and have served as a nutrient-dense, sweet treat for all of that time. Don't vilify fruits or fall into trendy, far-fetched diets. You can easily make small changes to eat healthier by cutting refined sugars and choosing natural foods over the new artificial products. This is a small change, but makes a huge difference.

Life is too short to eat foods that you don't love, or that cannot satisfy your cravings. If your healthy meals are not super tasty, you won't be eating them for long! Adopting simple ayurvedic routines, sticking with the basics, and incorporating fruits can be delicious and fulfilling. Eating this way feeds your body, soul, and spirit. It makes you feel your best and supports a natural state of well-being.

BEAUTY COMES FROM WITHIN

Eat vibrant foods. Fuel your body with a rainbow of bright, colorful, and nutrient-dense foods. More than just nature's candy, your skin will naturally reflect your colorful nutrition. You radiate what you consume. Beauty, in more ways than one, comes from within, and choosing the right nutrition will show immense benefits. Discover all the creative ways to activate enhanced beauty, longevity, and luminosity through color.

In the pursuit of radiant health and the best quality of life, start filling your meals with colorful, plant-rich superfoods that make your body thrive. Add citrus to your water, colorful, bright veggies to your plate, and nature's herbal healings to your daily routine. With time, your body will start to crave these life-giving foods.

Aside from the delicious flavors of healthy foods, colorful foods are packed full of antioxidants, vitamins, minerals, and wellness benefits. Different nutritious ingredients promote healing modalities for the body. For example, leafy greens reduce the risk of heart disease, obesity, high blood pressure, and mental decline.

Don't contaminate your body and your mind through toxic food, unhealthy beverages, and harmful emotions. This doesn't mean to suggest that you need to abandon your favorite foods. Never deprive yourself of food that makes you feel good. Allowing yourself these foods will make this journey easier to sustain and hopefully be long-term. Additionally, do not be blinded by fad diets and the anti-sugar mentality. Don't allow yourself to be misled by mistaken belief. Social media has a great way of falsifying reality, and fad diets come and go. Your health is there to stay so long as you are willing to do the work!

Food offers immense healing power. Your health is your greatest wealth and *can* be within your control. By increasing your nutrition, you can help defeat medical conditions in a lasting and meaningful way, without medications and potentially harmful side effects. Use what nature has provided us to prevent, reverse, and cure symptoms. Treat your body right. We are not immune from illness, but we have control over what we consume, which can greatly impact our body's ability to prevent and fight illness.

LEVEL UP

Make a treat a ritual, and make it decadent. After all, nobody can stick to anything they don't enjoy. Life is too short to restrict your nourishment and your needs.

If you find food planning difficult or dull, find inspiration in the seasons and the weather. Every season brings new flavors, textures, and comforts. Try something unfamiliar. Practice with new herbs and spices to elevate your cooking. Try ginger, turmeric, mint, basil, oregano, or whatever is growing in your garden or out in nature. There is something magical about creating life in any capacity. Knowing that you have grown these amazing flavors yourself can make them even more enjoyable and fun.

Gardening is a great way to be more in touch with nature. Nature allows us to connect to something larger than ourselves. Gardening and cooking your own nutritious foods will remove the stigma of healthy foods being boring. Doing it every day, or as much as possible, gives you something rewarding to do and look forward to. You can sit back and watch your creations bloom to life and then take them to your kitchen table to enjoy. There is much more positivity to gain from real, whole foods. Spice up your plate and your palate with herbs. These luscious leaves—think parsley, basil, cilantro, mint, and the like—not only add enticing aroma, fresh flavor, and vivid green color to food but also have exceptional health- and skin-benefiting ingredients. You can make foods enjoyable by aligning them with your taste preferences.

NATURE'S PHARMACY: HEALING HERBS TO INCORPORATE INTO YOUR WELLNESS ROUTINE

Basil

The aromatic smell of basil is enough to make anyone feel good. It is an antibacterial superfood known to balance blood sugar and balance the effects of chronic stress in the body. There are many different types of basil, but the nutritional benefits are the same. It's an excellent herb for disease-causing bacteria. Its flavors are so robust it's hard to imagine the work it's doing while you enjoy it!

Mint

With phytochemicals, mint is great for digestion. Its aromatic hues can help fight nausea alone. An herb with natural cooling and anti-inflammatory properties. Add to your salads, smoothies, and beverages. Your stomach will thank you, and your skin will too!

Oregano

A mouthwatering Mediterranean flavor, oregano packs a powerful punch for taste and is a great antibacterial agent. Loaded with antioxidants, this is a great ingredient to highlight in your dishes when you are fighting any infection. Make pesto, and add it to your favorite dishes.

Thyme

A healing agent with a distinct, lemony smell, thyme is known to help fight bacterial and fungal infections and boost mood. It's great for sauteing and roasting.

Rosemary

A very distinct flavor, rosemary is great for cooking and seasoning. Rich in antioxidants, it has been shown to prevent allergies and suppress congestion.

Parsley

It's the ultimate liver detoxifier. Along with its wide flavor, it is packed with wonderful nutrients and rich in vitamin C and antioxidants that help reduce the risk of serious health conditions. It's easy to add to your diet because it pairs well with many recipes. Add it to your eggs, salads, dressings, and sauces.

Even small amounts of these leafy greens can provide big flavor and even greater disease-fighting antioxidants. Don't be afraid to try something new and find yourself coming back for more.

There is an inseparable relationship between the mind and the body. Imposing this enrichment-focused diet will soon become a lifestyle. The brain works by creating cravings. After eating a certain diet for six to eight weeks, your mind will naturally begin to crave those life-enhancing foods. A whole world of healthy taste opens up to you.

Having a holistic mindset throughout this book and into your eating journey will enable you to apply this guidance and nutrition tips to optimize your health. Fuel your brain, gut, and immune health with goodness. It is often the most basic things that have the deepest impact on our lives—like nutrition.

Health isn't about being perfect with food or exercise. Health is about balancing those things with your desires. It's about nourishing your spirit as well as your body.

DINING IN: THE CENTERPIECE

Going out for food is always fun. But not enough people learn to love to cook for themselves and their loved ones. There is something about enjoying a savory, home-cooked meal that just hits different. With so many flavors, multicultural cuisines, and amazing ingredients to choose from in the grocery store, it's now so easy to cook incredible meals at home, and it does not mean you need to spend an entire day in the kitchen. You can get similar pleasure by dining in at home. It feels truly unique and has that warm, homey feel.

Food is a social centerpiece. Some of our most memorable and important moments in our lives are made across the table. Whether it be a marriage proposal, a business deal, a gender reveal, family traditions, holidays, or time to catch up on everyday life, it allows time to connect with others and have valued time with those you love. Nothing rejuvenates the mind and body more than shared human experience and quality moments where memories are made. Serve up an unforgettable experience. Turn off the screens and enjoy life's *real* moments. Bring meaning to life's celebrations and foster special bonds and new memories.

Dining with family or friends can be a huge part of creating a shared feeling of connection. There is nothing more wonderful and fulfilling than sharing food with those you love. It is nourishment of the soul and the body. Not only is this ideal, but it is so important for mental well-being to nurture human connection. Social interaction is a key coping mechanism for mental strength.

Hosting people at your home around a gorgeous and inviting table setting creates unforgettable memories—whether it be the sound of laughter, the clink of wine glasses, or the scent of food fresh out of the oven. "When someone cooks for you, they are saying something. They are telling you about themselves, where they come from, what makes them happy," as Anthony Bourdain so eloquently stated. The effort you put into hosting is a precious way to show you care. It is a way to treat yourself as well as others, bringing meaning to celebrations and special bonds. There is something to be said about eating good food and relaxing with people that bring you joy.

Life is all about balance, and making time to value your loved ones through self-made settings is a great way to enforce that. Create special moments and unfading, indelible memories whenever you get the chance! If, and when possible, eating meals sat down with loved ones in a peaceful, prepared setting will not only bring happiness but balance.

If anything, being confined to our homes as we navigated our way through the worldwide pandemic transformed our appreciation of cooking, particularly accentuating the desire to bring a connection of a dining experience into our homes. Any meal, whether it be casual or for a special occasion, can be beautiful if you take the time. Elevate the experience of making or sharing foods with family and friends. Savor the taste, be present, connect with nature, and dine alfresco if the weather permits. There is something enchanting, yet nostalgic, when sharing your meals in an outdoor setting. Get outside whenever you get the chance. You will not be disappointed!

So, set the scene, enjoy the moment, slow down, and eat like the French. Pull out the place settings, the cloth napkins, the candles, and the flowers (from your garden if you can), and cue the music. You won't regret it!

THE STIGMA

Food is designed to be a comfort and a way to nurture your body. Certain ingredients can help ease anxiety, energize you, improve sleep, and improve your mood.

As well as controlling the way our body defends our internal functions, skin, and mind, it also acts as one of the primary ways we get to socialize with friends and family.

Yet, the stigma attached to eating healthy is that it is boring, dull, and strict. In the culture and times we currently live in, many are obsessed with dieting and food restrictions. Most people associate eating balanced foods with eating nothing but green, non-flavorsome foods. For many diets, it can be that way. But, if you make food a positive experience by spicing your foods up and making them fun, they will be more exciting to eat, and you will be more likely to stick with it. That way, it is not a diet but a lifestyle. In fact, healthy eating is the complete opposite of boring. If you make it that way.

Life is too short to worry about restricting what you eat. So long as you find a healthy balance, that's what matters. Learning to love your foods will allow you to be passionate about eating and nutrition. You will learn to love your body so much that you want to nourish it.

Your diet is what you make it. There is no fun in eliminating certain foods from your life. Just because there may be an unhealthy stigma attached to them does not mean you need to get rid of them to be healthy—especially if they are your favorite foods. So long as you eat a balanced diet, that is what counts. You can eat your favorite foods, just in moderation.

You don't want to just survive; you want to thrive! Listening to what your body needs is so important for enjoying your diet and making you feel your best. If you want pizza, eat the pizza. You should not feel guilty about enjoying something you love. Joy and pleasure are also medicine. Like anything, balance is key, and if you allow yourself the time to enjoy what you love, it will only add to your healthy lifestyle. All you need to do to eat beautiful is put into place a balanced, nourishing, and feel-good diet.

Eating well and healthy is simply what you make it to be. Adding color, flavor, and a twist to healthy foods can make them inspiring. It can completely change your outlook on healthy foods if you spice up your usual dishes with something different. Never skimp on flavor, as that is what makes "dull" foods fun and delicious. There is no reason to be lazy or boring with food. All of these beautiful and fun ingredients are out there for a reason, to be loved and enjoyed.

SAY NO TO DIETING—SAY YES TO LIFESTYLE CHANGE

You are uniquely you. Your quest for optimal health should be as singular as you are!

Stopping yourself from getting attached to food labeling and diet trends is one of the greatest things you can do for your mind and body. With social media today and the elixir of diet and wellness trends, it is too easy to become misled or attached to labels. Food, like anything, can be habit-forming, so why not make it something enticing, attractive, and irresistible; something to look forward to! Rather than restrict, enrich your diet and nourish your body with positive repetition. You don't have to be perfect to achieve health and vitality. Small changes over a long period offer lasting benefits for the most intuitive, flexible, and healthy approach. Focus on food quality, personalization, and not being too rigid.

Food is restorative and regenerative. One of the greatest cura-
tive food categories our bodies require is fats—healthy fats.
Monounsaturated fats and polyunsaturated fats are known
as the "good fats" because they are good for your heart, your
cholesterol, and your overall health. For too long, fat has been
vilified. Far-fetched diets that eliminate fat are not something
to admire. Our bodies need fat for energy, balance, and proper
brain function.

Embrace the healing power of good nutrition and eliminate
the negative stigmas attached to foods that offer the true
nourishment our bodies need. Try adding healthy fats at every
meal and start to notice how much more satiated you feel and
how much more energy you attain. Some of the healthiest fats
to fuel your body with are high-quality olive oil, avocado oil,
fatty fish, whole eggs, avocados, nuts, and seeds, such as chia
and flax.

In this nutritionally confusing world of food, it's easy to feel
overwhelmed. When it comes to diet, there is no one way of
eating or detox solution. To achieve optimal health and a happy
mind, you need to find a balance that works for you. Aim for 80
percent nutritionally enhancing foods and 20 percent foods free
of restriction.

Listen to your body. Enjoying what you crave or simply what
you want, in the moment, that is healthy. This will allow you to
stay on track with mindful and nutritious lifestyle choices. These
small changes can help you reach a balanced regimen of healthy
and enjoyable eating habits. Eat real food mindfully and enjoy
it. There should be only one overarching rule when it comes

to food: to establish better eating habits by eating more real, whole foods that you simply enjoy, focusing on the foundations of health. Adopt small daily strategies to replenish and make life-enhancing changes.

INTERMITTENT FASTING

A great way to change your eating habits and seek better health is through intermittent fasting. If this eating lifestyle is new to you, there are some things you should know. A lot of people find intermittent fasting (IF) useful for weight loss. The basic concept of IF is limiting food intake to specific times. Instead of restricting and limiting what you eat, the focus is on when you eat. Aside from the increased metabolism boost, there are many other amazing benefits that come with IF between fasting and feasting. Some include:

- increased brain and cellular function

- weight loss

- cholesterol regulation

- reduced inflammation

- heightened concentration

- increased energy

- cellular repair

By eating within a designated time frame, it allows your digestive system to rest, reset, and naturally detox. Ideally, you should let your body fast for at least twelve hours routinely. For example, if you eat dinner at 8:00 p.m., try not to have breakfast until at least 8:00 a.m.

Like anything, there are extremes. Always listen to your body and do what feels right. It is important to understand your personal health and bio-individuality. Everyone is different, and, for women, it is especially important to eat when it feels right during specific times in your monthly cycle. Pay attention to how you feel, and choose what works for you.

With time, try increasing your fasting window one day a week, and strive to fast for fourteen to sixteen hours. This does not need to be something you do daily. Adopt a basic strategy of time-restricted eating in some form. You should see how you feel and how your body responds. Remember, the healthiest option is invariably the one your body is asking for. The important thing is knowing what works for you, and knowing what works for you is intuitive—always listen to your body.

Intermittent fasting will introduce intuitive and mindful eating into your life. As dieting is, and should be, a thing of the past, fasting can help you be more mindful of what you eat. Restricting, counting calories, depriving, or skipping whole food groups is not necessary and not healthy.

Instead, you can change your eating habits, be more mindful of what you enjoy, and become intuitive about what feels good for your body. By being present and in the moment, intentionally pausing, you can better enjoy food and good company. These simple shifts in behavior can easily become habit-forming. The benefits will positively shift to your body and mind. It will help you to focus on your health, feel better about yourself, and make better choices when you eat. For instance, it might encourage you to stay away from any screens while you eat. You can learn to savor and appreciate what you are enjoying, and the opportunity to nourish your body or share a meal with someone you love.

CHAPTER 7

EAT BEAUTIFUL

"A healthy outside starts from the inside."
—Robert Urich

A BEAUTIFUL PLAN

Food is life-enhancing and a pathway to health. My personal journey involved encouraging an optimal diet at a young age. I discovered that food can change your life, your attitude, your energy, and your immune response. Through this book, I hope to encourage you to focus on a better foundation of health to optimize your lifestyle with real, whole foods, foods that are alive!

Eating a nutrient-rich lifestyle enhances focus and boosts physical and mental energy and performance, which are essential and beneficial for our health. Finding your favorite foods is the best place to begin. Write down a list of your first-choice healthy and nourishing foods before reading this. Maybe even note some meal plan ideas. Then continue reading this chapter.

Eating beautiful is all about helping you find new nourishing foods and ingredients to add to your list. This section is here to bring color, flavor, and goodness to your life. It will help you understand how to create balance, improve your mind, improve your consciousness, and make real changes.

The steps below will help you create a plan. It will guide you through a beautiful eating routine and help you notice improvement in your health and, ultimately, your well-being.

Eat Fiber and Prioritize Protein; Avoid Starches and Added Sugars

Food is 100 percent our fuel, and while we think we must enjoy eating, it's equally important to remember that everything we put in our body affects us. Fiber and protein will make us both full and satiated longer without feeling heavy or sluggish. Fiber helps to sweep waste from our bodies, keeping us feeling light, while protein feeds our muscles.

Eating the right fiber-rich foods and proteins is essential in preventing fatigue due to a lack of key nutrients. For example, carbohydrates are a top fibrous nutrient. Choosing good carbohydrates over bad ones is ideal for keeping up good health.

Good carbohydrates rich in fiber include quinoa, oats, buckwheat, fruits, and vegetables. These can be easily substituted for poor choices of fibrous foods, which include white bread, pasta, and starchy vegetables. Keep gluten to a minimum, if possible, but don't fall victim to vilifying carbohydrates. Never be scared to eat, especially when it comes to real, whole foods. You must enjoy your food to sustain a beautiful eating routine. The moment you start restricting what you eat, you will lose interest in eating nourishing foods. To sustain a healthy lifestyle, you need to enjoy it.

Carbohydrates are in more foods than we think. They are in fruits, vegetables, and drinks. So don't be afraid to eat denser carbohydrate foods like lentils, legumes, starchy veggies, and grains. They all contain carbohydrates, and they can be good for you. Carbohydrates are an essential nutrient that can be fibrous and great for sustainability. So, never deprive yourself.

Protein-rich foods are a lot easier to be aware of. Those typically include meats, fish, and eggs. Yet, protein-rich foods also include nuts, seeds, tofu, legumes, and beans. Again, choosing nutritious protein options such as fatty fish, eggs, and nuts are ideal for a balanced diet. These are all lower-fat proteins, which are more nutritious and better for the overall health of your body.

You can attain as much protein from plant-based proteins like tofu, legumes, and nuts as you can from animal protein. Many prefer plant-based options now. But, many aren't aware of the amazing health benefits and availability of alternatives. Don't shy away from plant-based eating, as it is now more sustainable and easy to follow than ever. More on this is to follow.

Eat with the Seasons

Eat mindfully, with pleasure, and with the seasons. Enhance your plates with seasonal foods for freshness, creativity, and variety of life!

When you eat, think of the seasons. You should fill your plate with seasonal foods to get the most flavor and satisfaction. This will make more meals exciting and diverse. Eating a variety of foods is a creative and tasty way to eat almost anything. If you eat by the seasons, it will stop you from getting bored with your food. Take advantage of seasonal options and make each time of year an opportunity to add something new to your repertoire.

Being aligned with the seasons also helps keep us more in tune with nature. It can inspire you to cook some new and exciting dishes. This will make your meal planning, prep, and cooking more appealing. Eating flavorful salads, fresh fruit smoothies, and summer-style foods will make those cozy soups and hearty meals more enjoyable come winter.

Making meals seasonally appropriate will help you diversify what you eat year-round. The same goes for eating in different settings which are seasonally appropriate. For example, dining al fresco during the warmer months will make those cozy dinners inside more special. Surrounding yourself with fun ways to eat will help you enjoy your food that bit more.

How you eat is as important as what you eat. Eat with a unique perspective in mind. Eat mindfully and eat with pleasure. Why do you think so many important moments in our lives are made across the table? Because food nourishes the body and soul. When both are nourished well, there is calm. Take advantage of that time around the table!

Live Plant-iful

Eat a plant-rich diet. Get to know in-season foods from the ground, high in antioxidants and big in flavor. Making a conscious effort to bring more plants to your plate will pay dividends in how your body functions and self-regulates. A nutritious and healthy diet full of plant-rich and nutrient-dense foods provides our body with the nutrients and vitamins we need to remain healthy. We understand that proteins are the building blocks of the body and have a huge impact on your muscles, organs, and hormones. Yet, many don't realize how big of an impact plant-based food can have on the body.

Plant-based simply means making a conscious effort to add more plants into your diet. Eating whole, nutrient-dense, and plant-rich foods will help you discover their healing and nourishing power from nature's vitamins. Consider it nature's pharmacy. Plants have a wide range of vitamins and minerals. They contain key nutrients such as phytochemicals, antioxidants, fiber, and soil-rich proteins.

Examples of plant-based foods rich in these are kale, spinach, blueberries, raspberries, microgreens, swiss chard, and sweet potatoes.

There is a distinct connection between what we eat and how we feel. So many people follow low carb diets and restrict some of the most essential nutrient-rich foods from their diets. I encourage you to eat nonrestrictive and inclusive! Eliminating plants because they contain carbs deprives your body of nature's most pure vitamins and minerals. Plant-rich foods are an enormous pathway to better health and disease prevention.

The simplest way of adding more plants to your meals is to incorporate them into your everyday dishes. For example, you can simply use various powerhouse super seeds to sprinkle on top of your breakfast, lunch, snacks, or dinner. Some favorite vitamin-rich seeds include chia seeds, hemp seeds, and flax seeds, as they offer protein, healthy fat, and are rich in omega 3 and 6. They are great blended into oats, yogurts, smoothies, eggs, and spreads, or topped on salads. This simple biohack is available to everyone and can easily be added to any enjoyable meal with no extra effort. Superfoods like this nurture your body from the inside out by elevating your natural vitamin intake. Finding ways to supplement with foods first is one of the most important and advantageous aspects of maintaining a healthy lifestyle.

Another great way to increase the use of garden-fresh plants is to add fresh seasonal herbs and microgreens to your plate. Cilantro, parsley, oregano, basil, thyme, fennel, and dill are great options to add to almost any savory meal. Not only do they add flavor, but they also add key nutrients to your meals. Herbs are also considered elevated biotics, which are amazing for your digestive system, detoxification, and enhanced immunity. They work by adding healing B12 vitamins to your body.

In turn, this aids in digestion and helps restore and balance your gut through natural detox. A healthy gut and digestive system prevents fatigue and naturally increases metabolism, helping you function at your highest level, both mentally and physically. Microgreens are considered nature's superfood, delivering a powerful dose of nutrients rich in many beneficial antioxidants. They are known to have higher nutrient levels than most mature vegetables. This makes them a great addition to any diet.

Like herbs, veggies work in the same way. Eat your veggies. Enjoy the color, flavor, and nutrition they add to your life. When it comes to our plates, stay as close to nature as possible. Make your diet as beautiful as the rainbow with fruit and vegetables. They are some of the densest sources of full-spectrum antioxidants you can consume. The more colors you can get on your plate, the better!

Nutrition Is Medicine

Many people have resorted to vitamins to supplement their diet as an excuse not to eat vegetables. No supplement can outdo what vegetables can do for your gut. If you start doing this, you will notice a difference in your gut and how you feel within two weeks, possibly even in just a few days.

Your immune system and inflammatory system are highly regulated by food. What we eat reflects how we feel. Use food as your pharmacy and try these anti-inflammatory foods to improve how you feel.

Top ten anti-inflammatory foods:

1. Leafy greens

2. Extra-virgin olive oil

3. Vitamin C-rich foods—kiwi, berries, peppers, oranges

4. Cruciferous vegetables—broccoli, kale, cauliflower, brussel sprouts

5. Fatty fish—salmon, tuna, sardines, herring

6. Green tea

7. Fermented and probiotic foods—kombucha, yogurts, kefir

8. Nuts and seeds

9. Vitamin A-rich foods—sweet potatoes, carrots, butternut squash (colors that represent the sun)

10. Zinc-rich foods—high-quality meats, pumpkin seeds, brazil nuts, legumes, shellfish, and grains

How to add these immune-regulating foods to your diet:

- **Veg out.** Add colors to every meal. Vegetables and leafy greens are powerfully healing foods. Adding more soil-rich plants and leafy greens into your diet will enhance your body with magnesium and highly essential minerals, which are vital for a strong and healthy immune system and are more powerful than any supplement you could take. A variety of vegetables can be considered an elevated form of biotics as they facilitate satiety and healthy digestion.

- **Spice it up.** Various spices add color to your foods and make them fun. They also have impressive antiviral and anti-inflammatory effects that can ward off illness and disease. Here are some examples: garlic, turmeric, ginger, lemon, mint, oregano, parsley, and cilantro.

- **Don't fear oils.** Healthy oils are good for you, and quality matters. Cook with something that is as close to nature as possible. Prime examples include olive oil, coconut oil, avocado oil, and grass-fed butter/ghee. Try switching it up to add a variety of flavors to your palate!

Add Superfoods

Superfoods are nutrient-dense foods. Some can be whole foods like fatty fish, olive oil, yogurts, and nuts, which I have already highly recommended for a beautifully balanced diet.

But superfoods can also be found in smaller foods and powders. Even just a spoonful of certain superfoods can offer incredible benefits. You can easily add these enhancements to foods like yogurts, oatmeal, and smoothies. Here are some of the best examples of powerful energy in a spoonful and what they can do:

- Bee pollen, with high antioxidant properties, relieves inflammation, boosts liver health, and strengthens the immune system.

- Flax seed, which is high in omega 3 fatty acids, helps reduce inflammation, works as an antioxidant, and helps support gut health and regularity.

- Hemp hearts—rich in omega 3 and 6 fatty acids—help reduce the risk of heart disease and high cholesterol, balance blood sugar, and improve inflammatory skin issues.

- Chia seeds are incredibly rich in nutrients and minerals; these seeds help reduce cholesterol, are a great source of fiber and protein, and improve bone strength.

- Coconut oil, which is rich in medium chain triglycerides (MCTs) improves brain function, helps burn fat, and helps you feel fuller for longer.

Superfoods are not just a great way to eat beautiful. But, they are a way to maximize your health. The best version of you can be achieved by adding superfoods into your diet. They add a little zing to your meals and your body.

To enjoy these superfoods, here are some ways to incorporate them into your daily diet:

Breakfast Ideas

- **Breakfast bowls.** Add chia seeds, bee pollen, and/
  or flaxseeds to your fruit, oatmeal, or yogurt bowls.
  Smoothie bowls are a great option for breakfast.
  You can get in many highly nutritious fruits and
  superfoods here.

- **Green juice or smoothie.** This is an opportunity to
  get creative and increase the absorption of plant-rich
  nutrients, all while balancing alkaline health

- **Superfood scramble.** Use any variety of veggies, plus
  spices, herbs, and organic, pasture-raised eggs. It's
  quick, easy, and delicious. Top with microgreens, a
  drizzle of avocado oil, and hemp seeds.

- **Chia pudding.** Chia pudding is simply chia seeds
  mixed with water or a plant-based milk of choice.
  Leave to set overnight in the fridge and enjoy it as
  your breakfast. You can add bee pollen, coconut oil, or
  more seeds to the top to boost your superfood intake.

Lunch/Dinner Ideas

- **Salads and grain bowls.** Add flaxseed or hemp hearts
  as a delicious, crunchy topping. Top with microgreens
  for an aromatic flavor and amplified nutritional
  benefit.

- **Hearty soups.** Hemp hearts and coconut oil can easily be added to a soup, whether this is homemade or bought fresh from the grocery store. You can blend it into a soup or add it on top for extra flavor and health. For enhanced nutrition, add an organic bone broth and maximize the health benefits!

- **Coconut oil.** Cooking your meal in coconut oil will help you easily consume it in your everyday diet.

Snack Ideas

- **Smoothie.** Enjoy a smoothie and blend it with bee pollen, chia seeds, and coconut oil.

- **Flaxseed cookies.** You can easily use flaxseed to bake delicious treats.

Keep these superfoods easily accessible in your kitchen. Add them to anything and everything. You can enjoy them in salads, oatmeal, cereal, yogurts, smoothies bowls, and more.

To maximize the number of superfoods in your diet, try incorporating these in at least two of your meals daily. This helps you achieve a more plant-based diet, and your body and your skin will thank you. Having a balanced diet rich in vitamins and minerals is especially beneficial for healthy skin, hair, and nails.

These superfoods are vitamins in a spoon. They work by increasing your metabolic digestion, your energy, and they support your heart health with omega 3s and 6s. These food sources are incredibly healthy and should remain an integral part of your diet.

Find Your Favorite Adaptogens

Ashwagandha, turmeric, maca, and rhodiola are the real power players. All are mood influencers that are known to help with depression and anxiety. They help balance cortisol levels, which are stress hormones. Think of it as a natural alarm system for your body. It works with your brain to control your mood. In high-stress situations, cortisol helps fight off fear instincts and lower stress.

They are called adaptogens because they can "adapt" to how your body works and feels. Whether it is chemically, physically, or biologically, they help moderate the body's stress levels.

Adaptogens will make you feel good in the same way food and exercise can. Therefore, finding ways to add them to your diet is essential. It is also simple. They can be used as powders, supplements, and teas and can be added to recipes for flavor and wellness.

But never replace foods with supplements. Implementing both into your diet is key, especially real food over supplements. Having both in your diet will maximize the benefits to your health.

Adaptogens can assist with many physiological responses. From your mind to your energy levels and immune system. They help reject stressors that attempt to enter your body. In turn, this rejection improves health.

Benefits include preventing stress-induced fatigue, maintaining energy levels, and increasing focus and concentration. The right adaptogenic foods and adaptogens can also help balance blood sugar and boost immune health.

Some adaptogens work for long-term stress on the mind and the body, while others work on acute and short-term stressors. Long-term stress adaptogens are ashwagandha and ginseng. These work to balance hormones. Hormone stress is a regular and uncontrollable bodily stressor. The release and buildup of hormones can also affect our minds. Controlling hormones can dramatically lower stress levels.

Acute or short-term stressor adaptogens are turmeric and maca. Both contain active compounds that work to fight fatigue and anxiety. Turmeric's main compound is curcumin. Curcumin is a known ingredient that elevates neurotransmitters like serotonin, which works to suppress anxiety hormones and stress levels. Acute stressor adaptogens can also improve energy, immune response, and memory.

It is incredibly easy to consume adaptogens and make your mind and body feel beautiful.

Superfood Your Drinks and Meals

Increase the number of superfoods and adaptogens in your diet, and you will start seeing and feeling the transformation.

Love Healthy Fats

As with everything in life, you can consume too much of the wrong food. So, consuming the right foods is key, especially with fat.

Fat makes you full, not fat. Fats, when eaten right, are much more fulfilling than high carbohydrate meals, especially if you are looking for something to satisfy you. The right fats can offer benefits and maximize your overall health, whereas unhealthy fats can cause poor health.

You may be wondering what exactly the "right" fats are. Look for monounsaturated and polyunsaturated fats. These are the ones that offer many health benefits. These healthy fats can help with premature aging, improve heart health, and support cell growth. They optimize your health and also satisfy you for much longer than bad fats.

We have a physiological need for fat; however, that does not mean all fats are good. Broadening your knowledge of fats is crucial, as many people mistake fat as being bad, processed foods. They are the complete opposite. It is all down to which fats you consume that dictate whether they are good or bad.

Focus on the fats you consume. Avoid the temptation to consume hydrogenated oils such as canola, soybean, corn oil, and grape-seed oils. Ensure you are eating fats that are good for you, that support healthy brain function, and fight inflammation. There are an incredible amount of healthy fat alternatives.

High-quality fats are the answer. This includes grass-fed beef, fatty cold-water fish, eggs, avocados, olives, and healthier cooking oils. This includes extra-virgin olive oil, MCT oil, avocado oil, flaxseed, and coconut oil. Nuts and seeds are also packed with healthy fats and make a great snack.

Eating beautiful is all about balance. So, mix up your fat intake and put away the marketed fat-free foods. Change up your fat options daily and get creative. Changing your meals on a daily or weekly basis will get you excited about what you eat.

Nourish Your Body with Pre- and Probiotics

Many assume that pre- and probiotics are very similar. While they are both great for your health, they play quite different roles.

You may be wondering: what exactly are the differences between the two? Well, probiotics are beneficial bacteria that live and are found in certain foods. Whereas prebiotics come from fibrous foods that our guts find hard to digest. Prebiotics eat this fiber.

Gut bacteria, sometimes known as gut flora, play a vital role in many bodily functions. Good bacteria help fight off invading bad bacteria. They can also help fight inflammation and promote a strong immune system, as well as offering mood-stabilizing benefits. Research shows that the gut and brain are powerfully connected. A study in *Frontiers in Psychiatry* confirms that probiotic bacteria are particularly beneficial in improving moderate symptoms of depression, alleviating anxiety, and restoring sleep.

Thus, eating the right amount of pre- and probiotics is essential for good gut and brain health. As much as supplements are a great idea to increase your consumption of pre- and probiotics, you can get enhanced benefits from eating certain foods.

Healthy balanced diets provide the best gut health. Whole, fresh, and nutritious foods are packed with pre- and probiotics.

Below is a list of **prebiotic** foods:

- legumes

- chicory root

- oats

- bananas

- berries

- artichokes

- asparagus

- garlic

- leeks

- onions

Below is a list of **probiotic** foods:

- sauerkraut

- kimchi

- kombucha tea

- kefir

- coconut yogurt

- fermented vegetables

Avoiding processed, sugary, and oily foods is key to improving gut health. Scientifically, eating more prebiotics induces the growth of good bacteria in our gut.

Also, avoid relying on supplements, as you will consume a greater amount of pre- and probiotics from foods. They are a good addition to any diet. But they do not offer the same concentrations.

Optimizing your gut flora will only do you good. Our microbiome influences inflammation in the body. So, adding these to your diet is essential for supporting a balanced, healthy gut and mind.

At first, these steps may sound like a lot. But once you have created a new eating mindset and begin implementing sustainable dietary changes, it will feel easier. Setting small goals for yourself to implement balanced foods, adaptogens, biotics, and more will soon feel like a lifestyle. It is so simple to optimize your health by choosing beautiful foods over "easy" ones.

Remember to be kind to yourself. Never restrict yourself or be harsh on yourself. Get rid of the stigmas attached to eating well and right for your body. And keep in mind that a negative attitude towards food is not good for your mind or your body.

A healthy eating routine involves what your body needs as well as what it wants. It is an essential ingredient. Learn to nurture your body through mindful choices. Also, appreciate that you are in control of it. After all, only you can control your life and practice living beautiful.

Having the right tools makes cooking so much more enjoyable. Whether you use them to make your energizing superfood smoothie, to froth adaptogens in your morning coffee, or to mix your favorite pestos and salad dressings (with herbs from your garden...added bonus!), these items will make the process fun and effortless:

1. Juicer

2. Food processor

3. High-speed blender

4. Electric frother

5. Mixer

Having these healthy staples in your pantry makes it easy to assemble fresh beverages and meals. Improvised salads and grain bowls are even easier to make when your pantry is stocked with the ingredients to make a fresh vinaigrette or marinade, and when you have nuts and seeds to sprinkle on for an added crunch. These are some of my favorites that I use regularly. The guilt-free, aromatic flavors and multifaceted health benefits never disappoint!

Beautiful Pantry:

1. Oils and healthy fats: flaxseed oil, coconut oil, olive oil, avocado oil

2. Vinegar: red wine vinegar, apple cider vinegar, champagne vinegar

3. Condiments and seasonings/herbs and spices: turmeric, cayenne pepper, ginger, miso, etc.

4. Natural sweeteners: honey, maple syrup, coconut sugar, brown sugar

5. Nuts, seeds, and dried fruits

Beautiful powders, tinctures, and superfoods:

1. Chlorophyll drops

2. Trace mineral drops

3. Spirulina

4. Bee pollen

5. Turmeric

6. Nutritional yeast

7. Collagen peptides

CHAPTER 8

BOOST YOUR IMMUNE SYSTEM

"Wellness is the complete integration of body, mind, and spirit–the realization that everything we do, think, feel, and believe has an effect on our state of well-being."

—Greg Anderson

GET A BOOST

As much as eating healthy and introducing nutritious foods into our lives can improve our health and offer us well-being benefits, there are more benefits you can obtain from foods. Particular foods can boost your immune system, which is critical, as the immune system is the body's main defense mechanism.

When your immune system is in a healthy condition, you probably don't even notice it working away to protect you around the clock. However, you'll know when there's something wrong. As your immune system is your body's built-in defense structure, it helps protect you from illness and infection.

When it comes to our health, there are no quick fixes. But, we can make changes now that will support our immunity and pay dividends in the long run.

The world of wellness can be overwhelming and ever changing. With new trends emerging each day, it can feel like too much information, and we often feel obliged to give in to all of these trends. If your friend is trying something, you feel the need to try it too. But, your body will benefit from the foods and nutrition it enjoys and thrives off of. Instead, your body would appreciate it if you kept things simple. Go back to basics and focus more on the simple and wholesome foods that offer you optimal living.

It may feel silly to you to scrap all of the new food trends you have tried over the years. But, our bodies function best with natural foods that offer nothing but nutrition and health. It's okay to take a step back to attain the best health you can. Our wellness is dynamic and always in process, and our wellness journey is never done.

We must remember to focus on our wellness and life's quality at all times. Our wellness impacts our health. Our health impacts our life. To maintain your wellness and optimize your health, you can boost your immune system and protect your body and life from illness and age-related disease.

As mentioned in the previous chapters, our health refers to physical, mental, emotional, and spiritual well-being. As Ed Northstrum notes, "It's no coincidence that four of the six letters in health are heal." While "wellness" aims to enhance our well-being. Health and wellness are not just the absence of illness but a lifestyle based on choices that create good health. Our immune system is vulnerable to internal and external stress. If you really want to feel good all the time, you need to create balance and be consistent. A healthy outside starts from the inside. Down days and treats are fine, so long as you show up for yourself consistently and be mindful of what your body needs.

Creating habits that help you build a healthy immune response will increase your body's natural defense mechanism. Your health and vitality are generated by your deliberate actions. Now, more than ever, focusing on wellness, including a strong immune system, must become a priority of everyday resilience.

FIVE WAYS TO BOOST YOUR IMMUNE SYSTEM

Number One: Eat Whole Foods

Food is part and parcel of our everyday lives. Consuming food is the thing we do on a daily basis that makes the biggest impact on our health. Making the right food choices can be life changing.

Food impacts our health in a myriad of ways, one being our immune system. To ensure our immune system is in good health, eating whole foods is a great step to take.

Food is medicine, and your immune system relies on this medicine to function properly. Nutrient-dense whole foods will maximize the health of the immune system, as opposed to suppressing it. I learned at a very young age that the foods you eat can change your life, your attitude, your energy, and your body's ability to heal. Staying away from sugar, hydrogenated oils, and processed foods and swapping them for more vitamin-rich foods not only make you feel better but will improve the health of your immune system.

Eating an abundance of fruits and vegetables will help you naturally sustain a vitamin-rich diet. Eating as close to nature as possible, out of the garden, for example, will better encourage you to eat a plant-forward diet. There is an added benefit to being outside in nature. Plant a garden or venture off to a farmers' market for fresh produce. Find enjoyment in color and nature's gifts. It will help you make better food choices that will directly impact your health. Not only is it rewarding to eat your own homegrown foods, but it is often tastier and more affordable. Try adding soil-rich foods to your plate. Don't be afraid to get dirty!

Each color of the rainbow should be present in your diet. Each individual color has its own health benefits, providing different nutrients. For example, green leafy vegetables are packed with vitamins, minerals, and fiber, but low in calories. Eating a diet rich in leafy greens can offer numerous anti-inflammatory health benefits, including reduced risk of obesity, heart disease, high blood pressure, and mental decline.

Some of these colorful foods even offer the body prebiotics and probiotics, which are important for your gut's microbiome. We can ingest foods that serve beneficial gut bacteria. Foods such as fiber-rich bananas, cultured yogurts, leeks, garlic, onions, artichokes, sauerkraut, and fermented veggies are abundant in prebiotics and probiotics. Eating these foods will help you physically and mentally flourish.

Nutrient-rich foods include more healthy fats, protein, and carbohydrates. We need to fuel our bodies with nutrients that offer us energy and a myriad of health benefits, including a strong immune system. Be intentional about what you consume. Remember to eat a healthy and balanced diet of foods that offer your body nothing but goodness. Your immune system and health will thank you for it.

Integrating these foods and learning what your body loves will remodel your mind and spirit as well as your body. Eating the right foods will:

- reduce inflammation

- improve gut microbiome

- enhance nutrient absorption

- balance blood sugar

- improve metabolism

- balance hormones

- promote natural detoxification

- decrease fat storage

- enhance sleep quality

Number Two: Take a Moment

Wellness is a state of mind. Although food is important, boosting your immune system and optimizing your health is more than just your diet. It is about your wellness practices and how you spend your time. It's not just how we eat or what we eat. It is how we live, how we think, and how we love ourselves. Think about all the benefits your commitment to wellness can add to transforming your body and mind.

A healthy body will heal itself. Set yourself up for a Zen start and commit to your wellness today by taking time for simple acts of pleasure. Redirect your energy and focus on the present moment. It could be as simple as savoring each sip of your morning coffee, breathing in some fresh air, or getting some sunshine on your face in the middle of a busy day. Create a mindset for a healthy, happy body, mind, and lifestyle. Take a moment to invest in yourself; transform your body and mind.

There is so much about today's modern life that makes it difficult to relax and enjoy. Your mind and your body need and deserve these small moments of gratitude and appreciation. If you allow time for restful and restorative moments, it will help keep your stress levels in check. Managing stress through these moments will help level out cortisol levels. Cortisol is a steroid hormone that naturally occurs in the body and helps regulate your natural immune response. When they are balanced, our bodies can better respond to stress, regulate blood sugar, and fight infections.

Stress can weaken the immune system. When we're stressed, the immune system's ability to fight off antigens is reduced. That is why we are more susceptible to infections in times of stress. The stress hormone corticosteroid can suppress the effectiveness of the immune system. Thus, practicing moments of self-care and managing your stress will enhance your body's defenses and benefit your immune system massively.

Having breaks and taking time to center yourself creates balance. A mindful balance is how we obtain wellness. Wellness is a state of mind, and getting there offers a treat for the mind as much as it does for the body and soul.

Setting yourself up with a wellness moment helps us obtain these treats. Finding time to steep a balancing cup of tea, slip into something cozy, take a bath, meditate, and indulge yourself with restorative skin care can help us restore balance and well-being. Remember, the benefit of getting healthier is to maximize what your body can do for you. Invest wisely and enjoy these balancing, self-indulgent moments.

Number Three: Movement

Self-care moments can also involve exercise and movement. Throughout my own transformation, I have personally recognized the power and importance of using movement as medicine. Movement is a method used to benefit the body and the mind simultaneously. Moving your body has impressive effects on the immune system.

Exercise allows immune cells to perform effectively. Any form of exercise increases blood flow, reduces stress and inflammation, and can strengthen antibodies, allowing the immune system to work better.

Exercise is one of the pillars of healthy living. But that does not mean the exercise has to be rigorous and stress inducing to be effective. Gentle movements, such as walking in the fresh air, meditating in the morning, or doing yoga before bed, are enough to boost the immune system, dampen inflammation, and build strength.

Number Four: Sleep Wellness

Sleep is the pillar of wellness. Without it, we are depriving ourselves of its healing benefits. The power of being truly rested can improve how you move through and approach life. A rested mind and body will help you make better life choices, from wellness practices to your mood and how you choose to live each day.

We can have wellness moments every second of every day—even when we are asleep. Sleep offers the mind, body, and gut healing powers. Our bodies need rest to regenerate and regulate our energy, from breaking down our food to resetting our brains. How you start and how you end your day plays a significant role in the quality of your sleep and your body's natural sleep cycle. One of the best ways to start is to stimulate your circadian rhythm with morning light, as it organically optimizes your body's melatonin for a better sleep ahead, not to mention the metabolism and mood-boosting benefits!

Sleep also has restorative benefits for the immune system. During sleep, your immune system releases proteins called cytokines. These cells can promote sleep. Certain cytokines need to increase when you have an infection or inflammation or when you're under stress. Sleep deprivation may decrease the production of these protective cytokines.

If you struggle to sleep well or enough, there are some sleep rituals that may help you improve your sleeping pattern. First, you should practice prioritizing sleep. No matter how busy you are, you need sleep to reset and function properly. One of the best things you can do for your immune system is to prioritize sleep. Seven to eight hours is necessary for the body to re-energize.

Create a sleep routine. End the day with ease. Creating a Zen atmosphere in your bedroom will help you relax and drift off into a peaceful sleep. Before going to sleep, try switching off your devices and do something that naturally calms you, such as diffusing scented oils, meditation, calming music, sipping something sweet, reading, or taking a candlelit bath. Creating restorative sleep rituals and taking the time to shift your mindset is an invaluable investment in your immune system.

Number Five:
Supplement—Immune System Boosters

Since the worldwide pandemic, the popularity of immune-boosting herbs and superfoods has reached new heights. With our minds and bodies under constant stress, we have an increased need for supplemental nutrients to support our health and well-being. Now, more than ever, we need foundational nutritional support. Finding ways to introduce holistic and homeopathic supplements into your life can have a pharmaceutical effect, strengthening the body's natural immune response. Understanding the key supplements to aid in strengthening your immune system and building physical fortitude is essential to cultivating good health. If we all take a step toward ensuring our sufficient intake of vitamins, nutrients, and minerals, we can boost our immune system and fight off illness and infection.

These supplements are known to have immunity-enhancing potential. But keep in mind they are called supplements for a reason, as you are using them to supplement your diet. The base foundation of your diet, your lifestyle, and how you manage stress plays a vital role in your immune health. Add nutritious food, regular movement, good sleep, and self-care rituals before you begin with supplements, which should be added as an extra benefit, not a replacement.

Some supplements to include for increased immune function are:

- probiotic

- zinc

- vitamin D

- vitamin C

- vitamin B6

- turmeric

- omega 3

- omega 6

- elderberry

- medicinal mushrooms

With these mindful practices in place, we can boost our immune system, we can obtain better health, and we can live beautiful.

CHAPTER 9

BODY BEAUTIFUL

"You are not your body and hairstyle,
but your capacity for choosing well.
If your choices are beautiful,
so too will you be."
—Epictetus, The Daily Stoic

WHAT MAKES YOU FEEL TRULY ALIVE?

Practicing creating and cultivating the life you want is crucial to your physical and mental health. Creating a balanced lifestyle is about more than just diet and exercise; it includes the all-encompassing power of nurturing your mind and body through natural movement. The ideal is to cultivate not only a lifestyle but a lifetime of benefits, maintaining the sweet spot between health, performance, and longevity. This balance is about incorporating everything that makes you happy, finding pleasure, and ensuring you make adequate time for it. Understanding the value of balance comes with understanding what makes you feel truly alive. Conditioning physical activities and movement directly affects your overall health, vitality, mental well-being, and longevity. Body movement of any kind can transform how you feel completely. Why not find ways to move and feel your best with a transformational approach to mind and body reshaping that's proven wholly necessary.

MANIFEST THE BODY AND THE LIFE YOU DESIRE

Exercise and physical activity are a vital part of a balanced and functional lifestyle. Movement is not only a great way to make you look good, but the increased endorphins you get from exercise alone can make you feel amazing from the inside out. The gains you unknowingly receive in applying physical activities directly align with your emotional health and well-being. Exercise of any kind can help you let off steam and clear your mind while dedicating quality time to needed self-care.

Finding movement and workout routines that you enjoy is the gateway to creating the body and life you've always dreamed of. While nutrition can contribute to your health and vitality, incorporating daily movement and endorphin-increasing activities can allow you to achieve a stronger body and mind, aligning your emotional health and awakening your spirit.

Since exercise offers immense benefits for the mind, you can also curate a well-balanced life. It helps more than just your muscles; when we feel strong physically, we tend to feel stronger in all aspects of our lives, constructing a calmer and more fruitful mind. The benefits are multifaceted as the resilience of your human spirit can be rewarded by the physical strength you gain!

FIND YOUR SWEET SPOT

When you think of working out and the most effective routines, it can be easy to feel overwhelmed. There is an abundance of exercise tips, advice, and routines out there. Don't let them consume you. You should go with what feels best for you. Every individual body is different, and not every exercise will satisfy you physically and mentally.

If you enjoy gentle yoga, so be it. If you like to break a sweat through cardio or HIIT, then go with that. Whichever exercise feels best for you is what you should go with. You should and will want to sustain lifelong exercise, so ensuring you enjoy it will help motivate you. You should feel excited to work out. Focus on your favorite exercises rather than counting calories or overtraining. You need to enjoy it to sustain it. Listen to your body and what it needs. Some days your body needs rest and recovery, while other days you can go the extra mile. How we move, how we eat, and how we think play a vital role in our health enhancement. Regular and even light exercise can improve your well-being in several ways. The most noticeable improvements are better sleep quality, increased energy, and elevated mood. Whatever your exercise regimen of choice, you will find it is the sum of the small efforts that make the biggest impact.

You can gain incredible results by applying physical activities that work on the inside and the outside. Aligning your emotional health with whatever workout feels right will awaken your spirit.

Working out is a mindful practice that pushes our bodies to the limit to become aware of what we as human beings are capable of. Being active affects your longevity as much as it does your current vitality. Getting into shape—being fit and active—is something we should all want to sustain throughout our lives.

Many assume the benefits of exercise are for the present body. The benefits go far beyond the current years. What you put in and what you do today affects the outcome thirty or forty years from now. There are incredible health benefits, and the work you put in now will benefit you in years to come. For those seeking weight loss goals, exercise can help you achieve those results quicker. It can speed up metabolism, improve mental health, provide clarity, and reduce the risk of health-related diseases.

GET ACTIVE

We often think we have to do much more than we need to in order to get the results we want. With little effort, the emotional result of getting active is instantaneous, and the physical result is far more rewarding not only in strength but in mind. After a workout, it is more common than not for a person to feel a sense of achievement.

If you are healthy, actively listening to your body, and ready to improve your fitness schedule, physical conditioning of any kind will always make you feel better. Moderate exercise a few times a week is more sustainable and provides you with a much healthier lifestyle balance than little to no exercise at all. Make time to fit movement into your day every day if possible. Quiet your mind and body through movement. Even twenty to thirty minutes of exercise per day can offer amazing health benefits and help you create balance in your life.

Wellness is all about consistency. Learn how to cultivate the lifestyle and routine that works best for you. Simply showing up to a class, your mat, or a walk outside every day is an achievement in itself. It is the tiny little moments where you show up throughout the day that sustain you. Those little moments will encourage you to have a healthy mindset and maintain a beautiful life in countless ways.

Become a fierce advocate for your health and beautiful life. Find ways to make physical activities enjoyable, natural, and refreshing. By adopting a healthy lifestyle that includes daily movement, you can boost your immunity and delay symptoms of aging and future diseases.

MOVEMENT AFFECTS MENTAL HEALTH AND IMMUNITY

Movement matters. Movement and physical exercise is our medicine. It does wonders for our physical self as well as our mental health. It is just as important to take care of your mental and emotional wellness as it is to take care of your body. It is not just for losing weight or hitting physical goals; exercise is amazing for feeling good. That feeling after releasing endorphins is like no other. Creating true well-being comes from being kind to your body and providing it with the nourishment to thrive.

Find the workout that best serves your mood, schedule, or energy level. Whether you enjoy high-intensity classes or gentle Pilates, all movements that involve strengthening the body and mind help us focus on the present. Studies show that movement can reduce anxiety and depression while regulating your stress hormone response, setting you up for a positive chain reaction to your overall well-being.

Movement and regular exercise help you get a restful and deeper night's sleep. With the benefits of reduced anxiety, you can improve sleep quality, feel happier, and activate your lymphatic system, which is ideal for repairing and recharging the body as well as boosting your immunity.

Movement improves our health as much as it does our physical appearance in intuitively feeling *body beautiful*. Vigorous activity is not always necessary to get things moving. Gentle movement, such as yoga, Pilates, or implementing simple bodyweight exercises is enough to incorporate into your daily routine and activate the lymphatic system. It is about understanding the most effective ways to put your body to work—for *your* body.

Activating your body's lymphatic system can have an amazing impact not only on your beautiful body but on your inflammatory response and immune health. This is highly beneficial for reducing and preventing illness. Incorporating a regular body regimen that induces sweat will activate your lymphatic system, aiding in your body's natural detoxifying method, which acts to clear toxins and fight infection. But, unlike the circulatory system, it can't flow by itself—it needs movement.

WORKOUT GOALS

Find out what works well for your body type and maintain a routine. One that suits your schedule and abilities. Become your own practitioner of your favorite or preferred physical activity. Whether that be running, yoga, spinning, circuit training, kick-boxing, dancing, etc. You don't have to be an athlete or exercise for a long duration. Do what you love and what makes you feel good, and do it well. Discover what your body craves, and find ways to incorporate it into your daily life.

Narrow down the exercises you enjoy most, and the ones you feel give you life. This will help you find the most motivating and beneficial workouts for you. Being in control of your own time and goals will also allow you to do what you enjoy and focus on things that make you feel good. The many benefits of movement are not limited to physical health. Exercise is one of the best ways to boost your mood, improve your mind, improve your consciousness, and make real changes.

Finding balance with your favorite exercise or workout routine will maximize your health and happiness and bring out your best self. We all know we should exercise. Research shows that people who move regularly have happier lives, more positive relation-ships, and manage depression and anxiety better.

At any chance, get outside and amplify your results! The fresh air is great for the mind and helps you appreciate life more. Being in nature has a significant impact on your brain, mood, physiology, and well-being. Spending time outdoors can be healing and beneficial to the body and mind. Surround yourself with nature by bringing your mat outside, going for a run, bike ride, or simply walking at any chance you get!

Take a moment to define your goals. Make them specific so that you know what you are aiming for. When you actualize your goals, they will feel more realistic to achieve. Whether you aim to be more flexible or to be able to do a headstand in yoga, writing it down will encourage you to keep going.

RECHARGE. REPLENISH. RECOVER.

If you have overworked yourself and you are fatigued, rest comes first. Rest days, when needed, are just as crucial to maintaining your physical and mental strength. You gain major benefits as you begin to consciously use your awareness by paying attention and becoming in tune with your body.

Health should be your number one priority. Therefore, days off are as necessary as days on. Days off will help with muscle recovery. After sweaty workouts, your muscles will need rest to recover and replenish fully. Days off are a good opportunity to nourish your body with vitamins, nutrients, and the self-care your muscles need. Again, it's all about creating balance.

For exercise and rest days, there are many ways to take good care of your body:

Step One:
Feed Your Body with Essential Nutrients

To get the most out of muscle training, you need to feed your body the right foods. For your body to recover from physical activity, it needs essential vitamins and nutrients. What you feed your body will enhance strength, mindfulness, and endurance.

Don't be afraid of carbohydrates. These can be highly beneficial for boosting your energy and glycogen levels on rest days. Rely on complex carbs such as whole grains, legumes, high-fiber fruits, and a wide variety of colorful vegetables.

Protein is also essential for muscle recovery. Whether you are plant-based or not, there is an abundance of options. Fatty fish, lean meats, and plant-based proteins are the cleanest and most effective sources of protein for lean, healthy muscles and repair.

Your muscle and physical fitness are intimately linked to well-being. An exercise regimen that builds muscle has a holistic effect and a multitude of benefits. Training and treating your muscles with good exercise and natural sources of protein, vitamins, and minerals means they will return the favor in kind.

Some enjoy fasted cardio, which involves not eating for a set period of time before running, cycling, swimming, or whatever your chosen cardio activity is. Studies suggest that you can burn more fat and more overall calories twelve and twenty-four hours after an exercise session if you are in a fed state during the exercise session.

Eat your superfoods, proteins, complex carbs, adaptogens, and vitamins, and your body will thank you for it.

Step Two: Listen to Your Body

If something is on your mind, a great way to process emotions and thoughts is to let them pour out through physical activity. Listen to what your body needs, get up, get active, and sweat it out!

To keep up a physical routine, it truly needs to be enjoyed. For it to be enjoyable, your body needs to be able to cope, have fun, and feel good postworkout. Having a flexible perspective will lead to sustainable results.

If your body requires you to sweat more, do it. Increasing resistance training will not only improve your flexibility and overall strength but will also balance your focus. It becomes increasingly difficult to maintain muscle, balance, and flexibility as you get older. Perpetually training your muscles as you age contributes to better balance and enhances your quality of life.

High-intensity exercise, from cardio to muscle training, has impressive results for longevity. Your body will benefit in future years from improved flexibility and mobility.

If you prefer gentle exercise, this can have similar effects. Strength training keeps your mind and body young. Slow movements, such as yoga and Pilates, are known as eccentric training. It boosts your mood and builds strength. The increased energy you gain from gentle movement is life-enhancing.

CHALLENGE YOURSELF

From time to time, it is good to challenge yourself. Strive for an unimaginable yoga pose, distance run, or better yet, learn how to do a split. You may find a new activity you love. Or even better, your mentality will expand and feel good from trying new things.

It is never too late to start exercising or to try something new. Develop a growth mindset. Anyone can create new habits at any given time. Time is your virtue. Thus, being consistent and making time for exercise is the key to moving in a healthy direction, and has been shown to increase health and happiness.

INVEST IN YOURSELF

Being fit does not define one's worth. However, the act of caring for your body is an investment in yourself. Find a good balance of exercise that works for you and your body's needs without overdoing it.

Caring for your body in a way that you define for yourself can strengthen the connection you have within. It's never too late to rejuvenate your health routine. Be curious and keep an open mind. Everyone can create new habits at any given time. You just must be consistent.

As you begin any given activity, it may be a great time to set the intention with an affirmation such as "I am an athlete" or "Today my body will become stronger." Telling yourself you are capable will create a catalyst to push you through and reaffirm you can succeed.

It's not about perfection. It is about effort and how you show up for yourself. Exercise and wanting to feel your best should be redeeming and for your own benefit. Too many of us are attached to physical stigmas and idolize others for looking a certain way. A beautiful body is one that you are happy with, not a body for the sake of pleasing others or for social comparison. The most important thing is to stay strong, so you can do the things you love to do for a lifetime.

Exercise, like all other lifestyle factors, is your choice. It is only you who can cultivate the life you want to live—whether that means having an equal balance between things that make you feel good or prioritizing certain things. Balance is about what makes you feel, look, and want to do good. It is the single most important thing we can do to improve and maintain our health.

If you optimize your days on and days off, you will cultivate the body and health goals you have set out to achieve. It will allow you to create a connection within yourself. Exercise and routine are all about preference and listening to your body. Intuition will make your goals and mindset become vivid and help you sustain a beautiful way of living.

FRESH BODY, FIT MIND

Let's talk sweat and endorphins. Movement awakens our endorphins, which gives us sustainable energy for the day and alleviates responses to both physical and emotional pain. Body movement of any kind has the ability to transform how you feel. The great thing about exercise is that anybody can do what feels right for them.

Workouts and movement come in a variety of shapes, sizes, and strengths, and that's the beauty of getting physical. One day you might want to get hot, get sweaty, and burn away your stresses. Next, you might want to release mental stress by taking a brisk walk outside and breathing in some fresh air. There's nothing quite like the endorphin rush that comes after a sweaty workout. These daily adaptations not only boost brain power but improve your long-term health with positive change.

Whenever you're feeling stressed or overwhelmed, take a break and sneak a workout in or simply go for a walk. It does not have to be a long walk—even fifteen or twenty minutes of cardio can help get your blood flowing, your heart pumping, and your endorphins rushing.

Using movement as your everyday therapy is not only good for the body but also for the mind and soul.

If you have a busy lifestyle, worries and stresses on your mind, or need to let off some mental steam, a great way to process this is through physical activity. Exercise encourages mental clarity.

A great way to process feelings is to let them pour out through physical and/or creative activity. Body movement of any kind has the ability to completely transform how you feel. Any activity, from cycling, dancing, yoga, and Pilates to running and hiking, increases endorphins and serotonin levels in the brain and body. These hormones are both stress releasors and happiness chemicals that work to combat both physical and mental stress. These opportunities for movement can help release tension from the body and help sort out your thoughts. It also helps keep the mind and body focused on the present.

They help decrease tension and awaken the body and mind to a more positive attitude. This helps to boost energy and increase physical endurance. Not only will this improve your workouts, but it can also encourage you to work out more. Once you get that endorphin release, your body will crave it more and more. There is nothing quite like a rush of release once your blood starts flowing and your endorphins start pumping.

Your natural response to physical activity is exactly what your mind, body, and soul need to sustain a beautiful and healthier life.

GET HOT

Creating an active weekly routine focused on getting up and moving will help you stick to it. If you get bored of the same routine, mix it up instead of getting bored and burnt out. There is an abundance of options for getting hot and active, from HIIT, yoga, Tabata, circuit training, running, and Pilates. In an ideal world, your exercise routine should consist of aerobic activity and resistance training. Even just twenty minutes of activity can elicit profound benefits.

All benefit the body in different ways, from lengthening to strengthening your body. Whatever your goal is, go with a workout that will fulfill that. You don't have to implement everything at once. A mix of different physical modalities will help you attain the best end results. When committing to an exercise regimen, the best workout is the one you will actually do!

BODY WORK—MUSCLE RECOVERY

Looking after your muscles and fascia is so important for optimizing your strength. Hence, rest days are vital.

Your fascia is the glue that holds everything together. It is the soft connective tissue found just below the skin's surface that surrounds every organ, blood vessel, nerve, bone, and muscle. Muscle and fascia make up the myofascial system, which can cause muscular pain and increase the risk of injury when damaged. It is important to keep the myofascial system strong to prevent muscle pain, discomfort, and tears.

There are a few ways to take care of your body, muscles, and mind on rest days, which in turn, can maximize your productivity, physical health, and mental health. If you are looking to take your body and workouts to the next level, active recovery and conditioning are an absolute must!

It can be overwhelming trying to incorporate many new habits into your daily routine. Simply striving to focus on one of these life-enhancing practices at least once a week as a moment of self-care is a great start.

Focus on these functional movements, activating cellular rejuvenation, and see amazing gains. Great things to practice or do on those days off include:

Stretching

Stretching alleviates tight muscles, increases flexibility and blood flow, and rejuvenates energy levels. Put on some soothing music and set a timer on your phone to dedicate adequate attention to the myofascial release of your muscles. Focus on your breath, elongating, and toning. Stretching causes increased blood and nutrient flow throughout the body, leaving you feeling rejuvenated and surprisingly energized. It also helps create long, lean muscles.

Roll Out

Foam rollers provide an easy way of having a myofascial release, which can help loosen fascia so that chronic pain, digestive problems, and injury can be resolved. This can aid in reducing muscle soreness and improving range of motion for future sweat sessions. Foam rolling also helps with lymphatic drainage, which means that fluid buildup around your muscle gets broken up, allowing you to move better. Foam rolling oxygenates the blood, which will hydrate the fascia, activate your lymphatic system, help to create movement, and flush the buildup. A perk of this sometimes-painful foam rolling session can also include the decreased appearance of unwanted cellulite!

Yoga

Illuminating is so much more than stretching! Yoga is great for the mind and body, relieving physical and emotional stressors. Much like cardio, practicing yoga comes with a long list of benefits to the body beyond fascia. It can improve your flexibility and balance while simultaneously increasing your strength. Making time for these sessions is not only good for your body, your muscles, and your physique, there are also mental health benefits, like lowered stress and anxiety.

Epsom Salts Bath

These bath salts contain magnesium sulfate, which promotes muscle relaxation and helps to prevent aches, cramps, or tight muscles. The simple act of soaking in warm water can help relax your body and reduce exercise-induced muscle soreness. This genuine relaxation and physical self-care moment can have a positive ripple effect on your overall well-being, setting you up for a better day ahead.

Fascia Blasting

It helps to loosen the fascia, which helps muscle soreness, and can give the skin an appearance of being firm. The benefits of improved recovery time from workouts and enhanced muscle tone are worth the increased massage stimulation. This type of bodywork can facilitate the stimulation of your lymphatic system, promoting the flush of toxins from your body.

Deep Tissue Massage

Massages are an amazing treat for lingering tight and sore muscles and flushing the body of toxins. I recommend drinking plenty of fluids before and after any muscle work to stay hydrated and obtain the most beneficial results.

Making time for down days and the above things will not only improve your body, muscles, and physique, but will also help mentally with stress and anxiety.

Cold Therapy

Chill out with deliberate cold exposure. While this may not sound appetizing, you will be surprised at how your body craves the benefits that ensue. Use cold to recover, whether it be an ice bath, cold shower rinse, a whole body cryotherapy session, or a cool but refreshing plunge. Start small, and

access your discomfort using uncomfortable but safe tempera-
tures. The best way to explore this is by exposing yourself to
cold for a few seconds and increasing each time to test your
resilience and increased mental strength that comes along with
it! Used for health and performance, these can all come at no
cost but reap major health benefits, aiding in muscle recovery
and mind management. Try using your breath to stabilize and
calm your nervous system. The benefits are known to speed up
metabolism, reduce inflammation, and improve sleep, focus,
and immune response. You will be surprised by how much your
previously aching muscles have relaxed and your newfound
vitality.

Get Heated

The therapy of using cold exposure and then heat exposure is
said to be great for activating your lymphatic system—your
body's natural detox center. Sweating is one of the healthiest
ways to detox and restore your body, and it can also be a great
self-care moment.

Saunas, infrared, warm baths, and red light therapy are all amazing sources for restoring health in the body and mind. Heating
and detoxifying improve the immune system, alleviate pain, and
enhance circulation. Use this time to stack your healthy habits.
Meditate, breathe deeply, and make sure to refill your citrus-in-
fused water and hydrate! Bonus: add your trace minerals drops
for added hydrational benefit.

Own the Moment

Feel good and find balance. Feeling good before working out is a great motivator. Be intentional. Liberate yourself from what holds you back. You are entirely up to you. Be empowered to see the world as your stage, to try new things, and make every moment count. The most basic things in life can make us feel good. Make a stronger, more capable body today. This can be achieved in several ways. Starting the day with a positive mindset through meditation, natural light, and hydration is a great place to start. This improves focus, energy, and mood.

Your body is constantly sending messages to your mind. Meditation and morning stretching are great ways to practice alignment. Alignment helps with good posture. It lengthens your spine and alleviates back pain and pressure on your central nervous system. Good posture can give you more energy and help lower stress. Holding your body aligned and your head up throughout the day is a good self-motivating technique. Look up. Be proud of your journey and the activity you are about to embark on before each exercise. Bring purpose to your mat, run, or chosen activity.

IT'S YOUR TIME—BE STRONG.
BE BEAUTIFUL. BE YOU.

When you feel good, you look good. When you look good, you feel good. Your routine should inspire you to look in the mirror and say, "I'm ready to conquer the day!" This is your moment to feel confident in your own skin. Dressing for your workout can boost your motivation that much more, as can good equipment. If a workout is part of your daily routine, use it as an opportunity to get creative and inspired. Use this as an element to infuse little luxuries into your every day. Whether it be comfort, color, or sustainability, be inspired. Find what motivates you, and put your best foot forward to help you achieve just that.

Much has been made of the serotonin-boosting appeal of dressing up—why not do it for your physical fitness routine? Attire can offer a glimmer of escapism, even while remaining homebound, and it doesn't need to break the bank. You don't need much to get a good workout at home or at the gym, but these tools can make it a little more fun. Get ready to channel your inner athlete.

Must-have gym essentials:

- comfortable exercise clothes

- supportive sneakers

- resistance bands

- yoga mat

- glass water bottle

- gym bag

- workout gloves

- wireless earbuds

- microfiber gym towel

- sliding discs

- ankle or wrist weights

- bosu or balancing ball

Recovery tools:

- foam roller

- CBD muscle recovery

- Epsom salts

- Theragun

- massage ball

- stretch bands

Find inspiration from others that gives you the innovation to prepare you for physical activity, but do not compare—the aim is to feel good. It's important to look after our physical body for numerous health reasons, but not obsess over it. The ultimate goal is to feel your best, and that starts from within. You are powerful beyond measure!

CHAPTER 10

GIVE BACK

*"If you restore balance in your
own self, you will be contributing
immensely to the healing of the world."*
—Deepak Chopra

ONE SIMPLE ACT

It's time to do the work. There is no greater time to make a difference than now. Believe in yourself. Do your part now and forever. The mindset you approach your life with makes all the difference. Through the lifestyle tools you have begun implementing and mastering, you can share your knowledge when you choose to live beautifully, through one simple act of kindness—giving back, acting now, and making an impact in the world—understanding that small and simple acts of kindness and encouraging behavior can make a huge difference and will help us lead the way to a healthier and happier world.

Contributing to something beyond oneself is a powerful mood enhancement. The idea of giving back goes hand in hand with how simply feeling gratitude can have far-reaching benefits—it's a kind of mental vitamin for the soul. There are countless ways to improve one life, including your own! Give yourself permission to do good in this world not only for others but for yourself! Connect to a deeper sense of purpose.

Your health and your presence in this world should never be taken for granted. That is something I discovered throughout my tumultuous health journey, and this realization is something that I carry into everyday life with me. I hope this book encourages you to overcome some of life's challenges and realize your full potential. I chose to spread awareness and help others living with compromised health. What I learned along the way was that there is much more than our health alone that is compromised, and sharing this outreach to help others became abundantly more profound and impactful. There is an opportunity, after hardship, to rebuild in a better way, producing a rare chance to push ourselves to a new level of consciousness and empathy, being intentionally present.

MY DREAM

My dream isn't just to help myself achieve ultimate health and wellness; it is to make a healthy lifestyle achievable by all—one where you can tackle future challenges and respond effortlessly. My relentless dedication to wellness and living a quality life is not only for myself but for those I choose to share my life with. Part of my DNA is to motivate and inspire others to live their best, healthiest, most beautiful lives where all the ingredients come together. I feel strongly that finding a sense of purpose and meaning by helping others can be the catalyst to help do just that! You will be doing something good for yourself while doing good for those around you.

For me, if sharing my story helps just one person, then it will have all been worth it. I believe in generosity. The more you give, the more you receive. We all need to express gratitude and humility.

We will all go through challenging times at some point in our lives. It is the mindset with which you approach life that can make all the difference. As you now understand, the most important changes you can make are lifestyle related. With the tools and health habits you utilize throughout this book, you should build mental and physical resilience to handle life's obstacles as they come. My hope is that you feel empowered to make lifestyle changes and effectively improve because you can. Life is filled with a variety of events that we simply have no control over. We cannot always change our circumstances, but we can change our attitude. You are capable of influencing the direction of your life. You can control how you experience the challenges of life. Elevate your perspective. Exercise your curiosity. Take ownership over your health and your life. Enjoy the journey as opposed to always focusing on the destination. Choose to spend your time engaging in activities that mean something to you. Make a commitment today to learn new things that open you up to new experiences. Try seeking the upside in every situation and make everyone feel good just by being you. The sooner you can attune your spirit to that idea, the easier and happier your life will be.

The thing with health and lifestyle is that it doesn't come naturally to some, especially since the boost in false advertising and nonnatural ingredients has become the norm. Many believe that to achieve ultimate health and wellness, you need to do so much or eat a certain type of new food or fall into a trend. When, in fact, the most achievable and effective way to better health is stripping it back to basics and motivating self-behavior. Adhering to smart lifestyle choices can make all the difference. Remember, the benefit of getting healthier is to maximize what your body can do for you.

YOU ARE ENTIRELY UP TO YOU

As much as this book can encourage you, it cannot make you do anything. You are the creator of your life. Therefore, it is essential that you consider these tips, put them into practice yourself, and hopefully encourage others to go on the journey with you. Expand your horizons. Enhance your ability to be more present. Find ways to repurpose the time you already have. Ask yourself, how can I serve myself and others? The gifts you give can be imbued with your presence. By simply being you and making a concerted effort to live beautiful, you can enhance your presence in the world as a genuine, authentic human. An air of humility always works well.

THE MOST IMPORTANT SKILL OF ALL: HOW TO LIVE

Once you have done some of the inner work and given back to yourself, you can better foster your ability to give to others. Be extraordinary in the ordinary. Get involved. Beauty is an expression of the soul, not the ego. There is an inseparable relationship between the mind and the body. Having relentless dedication with your attitude towards a healthy and abundant life will make for overall health and wellness and help you learn how to live fully. It will help you discover a newfound appreciation for the simple pleasures in life.

A newfound attitude for learning how to live and be healthy will help you cultivate new action patterns and attain real results, which will have long-lasting effects on your overall health, well-being, longevity, and prevention of age-related diseases. Overall, it will help you to live more beauti-fully.

Reading this book should inspire you to act now to attain results—ones that can last a lifetime. Likewise, I hope it gives you the energy and motivation to encourage others to come together and make a difference in each other's lives.

These new practices and life lessons will transform you into a student of human nature, which we all should be, and you will demonstrate your ability to create profound change through one simple act of kindness. It is a really meaningful way to discover how good it feels to give back.

Always lead with love, proudly standing at the forefront of change. Love is essential to making yourself and others around you more vibrant and confident living in a world full of possibilities. It is when we choose to venture beyond our routines and expectations that we can enter a new world of experiences. Likewise, it helps to elevate your perspective in life, especially when you give back. There is great reward when you can nurture your inner life and those around you.

EXPAND YOUR MIND, EXPAND YOUR LIFE

Human connection can draw you to the fullness of life as much as it can expand your mind. Not only will it intensify your experience with life, but it will also foster deeper development of empathy and intensify human connections while improving your creative powers. This deeper empathy will give you temendous momentum, which helps you appreciate every life moment and life encounter. It precipitates an intense appreciation for life. You really never know what someone is going through. Understand that everyone has their own challenges, and simply being kind to each other can help make the toughest of times more bearable.

Through giving back and helping others, you can optimize your health and nurture your inner life. The enhancements that you and those around you will achieve will shift your world and help you discover the greatness of cultivating your life, being healthier, and improving your sense of gratitude.

Like other highs in life, the feeling of giving back and doing something purposeful for someone else can be addictive. When you appreciate life itself, the experiences are more intense. There is a power in interactive giving. Gratitude is a kind of medicine. This addictive craving will soon become a natural practice and part of your everyday life, which will have a ripple effect and encourage the world around you to be kind and give back too.

GIVE BACK

Spreading this awareness and helping others with compromised health is something that I found can have immense benefits. Helping someone can cost you nothing and benefit you both greatly. These benefits are invaluable, and there are so many ways that you can help someone else out. Be intentional with your thoughts and where you focus your energy.

SO, WHAT'S NEXT?

The next step is to reach out to someone with compromised health, or identify opportunities to give back to your community. With countless opportunities to help at no cost at all, the benefits are invaluable. Once you do, you can make an impact on so many people's lives for the better.

Although you can help in several ways, it is a good idea to start where your passion resonates, whether that be healthcare, children, education, mother nature, food, learning, or simply donating your goods to those who need help.

Put a plan into action. If you have a full-time career and a family to care for, you don't have to make these moments long-term. They can be short-term commitments yet still have a significant impact. There are easy ways to make a difference. Often the simplest gestures go a long way. Remember, you are the change agent.

The real results that will have the most lasting effects are in lifestyle choices. This enhanced care for yourself will transpire to caring for others, which will benefit your mind as much as your body. You are the only one who can make a change in your own life and create these sustainable differences.

Acknowledging your internal power and bettering your own health, energy, diet, and lifestyle will soon enhance your care for others. Being happy and healthy yourself can be a launchpad to motivate others to pursue happier and healthier lives. You will discover the power in health and gratitude, which will make you want to make others' lives as beautiful and as powerful as your own. The sooner you can attune your spirit to that idea, the easier and happier your life will be. When we give back, the primary goal is, of course, to make a difference in someone else's life. But the benefits of giving extend to the giver too!

There is no time like the present to harness the power to help yourself and those around you. Whenever possible, anchor yourself in the present. Appreciate every moment and every life encounter. Doing something small for someone else can benefit you more than you think. It is a lifestyle shift, and it will take up some of your own time, but it is so worth it. You are the change agent, and harnessing this power and sharing it with the world will make such a great impact on the world we live in and the spirit you carry through life.

Learn to look for fullness in every moment, and it will soon become an intention that rises in the body naturally. Implement these intentions and learn to live in the present. After all, it is the only moment you have.

CHAPTER 11

LIVE
BEAUTI-FULLY

"Though we travel the world to find the beautiful, we must carry it with us, or we find it not."
—*Ralph Waldo Emerson*

NOW IS THE TIME

Today is the day to remodel your wellness. Make small changes that will positively affect the rest of your life. Take charge and anchor yourself in the present moment. There is no better time than now to start feeling your best. Be proactive about your long-term health and well-being and how you choose to flourish in life. The choices we make directly impact the quality of the life we live. No one can do it for you. Make a conscious effort to take control of your health today.

As we come to the close of *Live Beautiful*, this is a reminder that this book is not a diet, not a cleanse, and not a tool to be strict. Instead, it is a lifetime resource meant to teach you sustainable, healthy habits to introduce in your life now and to take with you into the future. True and lasting change without restriction allows you to spend more of your time feeling your best self. How you eat, how you move, and how you feed your soul benefits your physical and mental well-being. Allow these self-care efforts to create more freedom in your life—full of possibilities.

When you master these habits, which will come with more practice, the benefits will serve you for a lifetime. You will be able to reap these healthful wellness rewards indefinitely, should you choose to make the commitment to yourself. Incorporating any of these wellness modalities offers inexpressible qualities that amplify all aspects of your daily life.

THE PILLARS OF WELLNESS

Being a practitioner of functional wellness myself, I wanted to share with you how to put the pillars of wellness together, and how they benefit one another. Eating beautiful, living beautiful, and feeling beautiful all come together to allow you to live an abundant life full of optimal health and enriched happiness. Through lessons I've learned and passionately studied, I feel compelled to share what makes me feel stronger, healthier, and truly alive.

If I didn't listen to medical guidance in my past, I certainly wouldn't be where I am today. No diet is a substitute for medical care. Learning to nurture and eliminate stress from your body and create a more healthy, balanced life is essential in healing any health condition.

My mission is to help people heal from the inside out, while incorporating daily practices and expanding appreciation for the interconnection in life. It has led me to places that I never thought I would go. I hope you carry out your dream to live a healthy and wholesome life. My goal is to better enable you to reach your goals and live a life free from restriction with vitality. Our health is our finest wealth, our greatest currency. We really must invest wisely.

To put into practice, you must attain the right mindset. Keeping your life and health in balance is an ongoing journey. Hopefully, by now, you understand how your mind, body, and soul can benefit from living beautiful. Though I hope you will turn back to this book many times in the future. Use this understanding as the motivation to accomplish what you want and achieve your happiest and healthiest self.

Forget the modern complexities of health. Stay committed, but stay flexible. Instead, strip things back to basics, which will help you live a simple yet rewarding life. The true tenets of wellness include good sleep, food, exercise, and good people. Surrounding yourself with the right elements will make a healthy life more fun and enjoyable. Embrace your capabilities. Keep an open mind, becoming more conscious of how you choose to spend your time and where you find enjoyment, growth, and connection to others.

As humans, we are often surrounded by harmful toxins without even realizing it. Everything from social media to diet trends can be toxic for our minds and bodies. Protect your peace and be intentional about what you consume. Curating a simple and personalized wellness routine can help you support a healthy mind and body.

The more you practice the essential pillars of wellness—nutrition, exercise, inner beauty, sleep, meditation, gratitude, and nature—the more natural it will feel for you. Doing things routinely and with intention will motivate your brain to receive the benefits.

STEP BY STEP

I invite you to start simple. Start small and create your own path to wellness by adjusting just one thing each day. Eventually, the tools in this book will come together, full circle, and help you create your own path to wellness. Sleep well, meditate often, practice gratitude, be in nature, eat right, and most importantly, live beautiful in every sense of the word. You have the knowledge, the tools, and the guidance to chart your own path. Learn it, live it, love it!

Embrace the imperfect and bring balance into your life. Foster a positive growth mindset for even the smallest of improvements—ultimately creating a healthy, happy life for yourself, your family, and your friends.

A final note. Embrace each day. Chart your own path to well-ness. Take life as it comes and remember to take good care of yourself. I want to serve you and help you live a beautiful life, one without restriction and one full of abundance. Most of us will live a long life; the question is: will yours be beautiful?

xx

Renée Marie

www.ingramcontent.com/pod-product-compliance
Lightning Source LLC
Chambersburg PA
CBHW020458030426
42337CB00011B/151